Selling to Hospitals & Healthcare Organizations:

A Glossary of Business Acumen & Personnel

Thomas J. Williams and Heather L. Williams

Published by Strategic Dynamics Inc. LLC.

Version Date 21050911

Book Design by Vanessa Maynard

Stethoscope by deliormanli. Stock number 5623147

TABLE OF CONTENTS

A SPECIAL THANKS   4

INTRODUCTION   5

PART 1: HOSPITAL BUSINESS & CLINICAL TERMS   7

PART 2: PART 2: HOSPITAL, PHYSICIANS &

   KEY HEALTHCARE PERSONNEL   174

APPENDIX 1: ACRONYMS & MEDICAL

   INDUSTRY ABBREVIATIONS   269

APPENDIX 2: ANATOMICAL

   ORIENTATION TERMS   278

APPENDIX 3: HEALTHCARE AGENCIES

   & ORGANIZATIONS   280

APPENDIX 4: PRESCRIPTION TERMS

   ADMINISTRATION METHODS—FREQUENCY   294

ABOUT THE AUTHORS   295

A SPECIAL THANKS

A special thanks to Robert L. Chatburn, MHHS, RRT-NPS, FAARC for spending countless hours reviewing this book and helping us define the correct wording for the various business and clinical terms and healthcare titles listed in this book. Rob is an expert in healthcare and is a noted author of several books and numerous articles published in peer review journals.

He is the Research Manager at the Respiratory Institute at Cleveland Clinic and he is an Adjunct Professor of Medicine of Case Western Reserve University.

INTRODUCTION

As hospitals migrate from a fee-for-service reimbursement methodology to payment for value, based upon patient outcomes; they are creating new business models and new relationships with insurers, physician practices, single and multi-specialty community clinics, ambulatory surgery centers, diagnostic imaging centers, specialized treatment service centers, specialty hospitals, skilled nursing facilities and other healthcare entities.

The hospital is now part of a healthcare continuum and this adds both an opportunity and a challenge for sales professionals that wish to sell their products, services and solutions. It's an opportunity because many sellers will be able to expand their portfolio within the growing organizational footprint. It's a challenge because new and different buying influences are evolving that speak a different language; often are in different geographic locations, with varying needs and requirements and who wish to buy collaboratively by soliciting input from others often within a committee structure.

To sell effectively in this new ecosystem today's sellers must understand the role and function of hospital and alternate site personnel and their language. We call this Business Acumen. Sellers that understand the language and business of hospitals receive immediate credibility, which is a foundation for building communication and trust.

This Glossary is designed as an easy-to-use reference. In Part 1 users will find Business and Clinical words that are commonly used within medicine, insurance, finance, supply chain and clinical research defined within the context of the hospital and their related entities.

Part 2 contains a Healthcare Personnel Glossary that describes the most common titles of hospital personnel along with a brief overview of their job. It is not an all-inclusive healthcare personnel dictionary because titles, roles and responsibilities often differ between hospitals of various sizes and within healthcare systems. In addition, there are differences in titles between community hospitals and teaching hospitals. The latter includes teaching titles and research titles which we deliberately did not add to this missive. Instead, we have provided the most common listing of job titles of personnel working within hospitals and associated healthcare entities. Because physician practices are being purchased by hospitals we did include those.

There are Four Appendices to assist the reader. Appendix 1 describes the most frequently used Acronyms and Medical Industry Abbreviations. Appendix 2 provides a short list of Anatomical Terms. Appendix 3 lists several Healthcare Agencies and Organizations that sellers may encounter in their discussions with healthcare personnel. Appendix 4 is a brief list of Prescription Terms.

We hope this glossary helps sales professionals improve their Hospital Business Acumen so that they can conduct better and more meaningful conversations with hospital and healthcare personnel and build great long-lasting business relationships.

THOMAS J. WILLIAMS & HEATHER L. WILLIAMS

PART 1: HOSPITAL BUSINESS

& CLINICAL TERMS

ABANDONMENT

The complete retirement of a fixed asset from service. This is usually after the removal of salvageable parts that can either be used or sold.

ABDOMINAL SURGERY

An operation that involves an incision into the abdomen.

ACADEMIC MEDICAL CENTER (AMC)

A group of related institutions that includes a teaching hospital or hospitals, a medical school and its affiliated faculty and other health professional schools such as a dental or nursing school.

ACCESS

An individual's ability to obtain needed health care services.

ACCOUNTABLE CARE

A concept to organize and deliver more proactive and preventative healthcare so that under ideal circumstances patients will have access to the right care at the right time.

ACCOUNTABLE CARE ORGANIZATION (ACO)

An ACO is a group of healthcare providers (e.g., hospitals, physicians, and others involved in patient care) that work together to coordinate care for the patients they serve. Under the ACO model they accept collective accountability for the quality and cost of care delivered to a specific population of patients that are currently enrolled in a traditional fee-for-service program. Within an ACO the patient is a partner in the care they receive. While ACOs began with Medicare patients, under the Affordable Care Act, all major payers are now offering varieties of ACOs. Today an ACO may be sponsored by physicians, hospitals or payers that coordinate, manage and provide care for patients.

ACCOUNTING

The art of recording, classifying, and summarizing in terms of money, transactions and events, that are financial, and then interpreting their results.

ACCOUNT NUMBER

The number created by a doctor or hospital to identify a patient for a medical visit and then stored in the patient's medical record.

ACCOUNTING PERIOD

The period of time for which an operating statement is prepared.

ACCOUNTS PAYABLE (AP)

The functional area of the hospital that is responsible for computing the patient's hospital bill and sending an invoice to the insurance company and/or patient. Also called the Billing Department.

ACCOUNTS RECEIVABLE (AR)

Assets that arise from services provided or the sales of goods to patients on credit.

ACCREDITATION

The process whereby a health care organization (hospital) is evaluated and determined to meet the quality-of-care standards determined by industry-derived standards established by an accrediting body.

ACCREDITATION SURVEY

The process used to evaluate whether a health care services organization meets specified standards for accreditation.

ACCREDITED HOSPITALS

The list of hospitals that have met the standards of the Joint Commission or other accrediting bodies for quality of care.

ACCRUAL BASIS (OF ACCOUNTING)

The method of accounting, whereby revenues and expenses are identified in specific periods of time, such as a month or year, and are recorded as they are incurred, along with any acquired assets, without regard to the date of receipt or payment of cash. This is distinguished from cash basis accounting.

ACID TEST RATIO

The ratio of cash, marketable securities and accounts receivable to current liabilities.

ACKNOWLEDGMENT

Any communication (electronic or physical) by a supplier that advises the purchaser that a purchase order has been received.

ACQUISITION COST

The total cost of purchasing an item. It usually includes the product cost and freight but may include time as well.

ACTIVE MEDICAL STAFF

Doctors that are members of the medical staff of the hospital excluding interns and residents.

ACTIVE SURVEILLANCE

This is a wait and see approach used by a physician to see if treatment may be needed because the patient may get better without the treatment. The length of time for active surveillance varies according to the patient's severity of symptoms, the risks and benefits of waiting, the progression of the problem, if not treated and the individuals age and medical history. This is also called Watchful Waiting.

ACTIVITIES OF DAILY LIVING (ADL)

An index or scale which measures a patient's degree of independence in bathing, dressing, using the toilet, eating, and moving from one place to another.

ACTIVITY BASED COSTING

A method that plans, measures and controls expenses associated with managing and monitoring the supply chain techniques for assigning cost in business processes and activities.

ACTUAL CHARGE

The charge(s) for a particular service/treatment by a health care provider.

ACTUAL COST

The purchase price of an asset.

ACUITY

Degree or severity of illness.

ACUTE CARE

Health care provided to treat conditions that are short term and episodic in nature.

ACUTE CARE HOSPITAL

Typically a community hospital that has facilities, medical staff and all necessary personnel to provide diagnosis and treatment of a wide variety of conditions including injuries to meet the needs of patients who require short-term care for a period of less than 30 days.

ACUTE CARE SERVICES

All of the coordinated services related to the examination, diagnosis, care, treatment, and disposition of an acute episode of illness.

ACUTE DISEASE

A disease characterized by a single episode of fairly short duration, usually less than 30 days, and from which the patient can be expected to return to his or her normal or previous state and level of activity.

ADDITIONAL DIAGNOSIS

Any diagnosis, other than the principal diagnosis, that describes a condition for which a patient receives treatment.

ADJUSTED ADMISSION

Hospital admissions that are adjusted to account for skilled nursing, chemical dependency, and outpatient activity.

ADJUSTED CASE MIX VALUE UNITS (ACMVU)

Hospital admissions, chemical dependency admissions, and births adjusted for skilled nursing and outpatient activity and for the hospital's mix of patients.

ADJUSTED PATIENT DAYS

Hospital patient days adjusted to account for skilled nursing, chemical dependency, and outpatient activity.

ADJUSTMENT

The portion of a medical bill for which a doctor or hospital has agreed not to charge.

ADMINISTRATIVE EXPENSE

An expense classification incurred in the general operation of the hospital, as opposed to the expense of a more specific department or clinical service such as rehabilitation services.

ADMINISTRATION

The department that includes the hospital CEO and his direct reports such as the COO, CNO, CMO, CIO etc. Their function is to develop an effective medical and support staff and to supply that staff with adequate equipment and facilities to provide quality health care to its inpatients and out-patients cost-effectively.

ADMISSION

Acceptance by a hospital of a patient who is to be provided with room, board, and continuous nursing service for the purpose of providing high quality cost effective care.

ADMISSION DATE (ADMIT DATE)

The date a patient is admitted for treatment.

ADMISSION HOUR

The hour when a patient is admitted for inpatient or outpatient care.

ADMISSION SOURCE

The physical site from which the patient was admitted such as a Home, Residential Care Facility, Ambulatory Surgery Facility, Skilled Nursing Facility, Intermediate Care Facility, Long-Term Acute Care Hospital, Prison/Jail etc.

ADMISSIONS

The number of patients, excluding newborns, accepted for inpatient care during the reporting period.

ADMISSIONS DEPARTMENT

The department where the patient is required to provide personal information and sign consent forms before being taken to a hospital unit or room. If the individual is critically ill or injured then this information is usually obtained from a family member. They typically manage admissions, discharges and transfers.

ADMITTED PATIENT

A patient that undergoes a hospital's admission process to receive treatment and/or care.

ADMITTING DIAGNOSIS

The diagnosis provided upon admission explaining the reason for the admission as stated by the physician.

ADMITTING PHYSICIAN

The physician responsible for admitting a patient to a hospital or other inpatient health facility.

ADMITTING PRIVILEGES

The authorization a governing board gives to a physician to admit a patient into a particular hospital or health care facility to provide patient care. Privileges are based on the provider's license, education, training and level of experience.

ADULT DAY SERVICES

Services provided during the day at a community-based center that provide meals and structured activities for people with cognitive or functional impairments, as well as adults needing social interaction and a place to go when their family caregivers are at work. These programs provide social and support services in a protective setting during any part of a day, but not 24-hour care.

ADULT INPATIENT CLINICAL RESEARCH CENTER

Care location for patients who have volunteered for National Institutes of Health-funded clinical trials involving investigatory drugs, devices and dietary studies.

ADULT STEP-DOWN UNIT

A unit within a hospital that provides a lower level of care for adult patients than an intensive care unit but a higher level of care than a typical medical-surgical unit. Sometimes these units are called Med-Surg, Medical or Surgical Step-Down units.

ADVANCE BENEFICIARY NOTICE (ABN)

Notice a health care provider should give a Medicare beneficiary to sign when providing a service the provider believes will not be paid for by Medicare.

ADVANCED DIRECTIVE

Written instructions recognized under law relating to the provision of health care when an individual is incapacitated. An advance directive takes two forms: a living will and durable power of attorney for health care.

ADVERSE DRUG EVENT (ADE)

An adverse event that involves the use of a medication(s).

ADVERSE EVENT-OUTCOME

Any occurrences serious enough to harm a patient during patient care. Some examples of adverse events are infections, venous thromboembolisms, pressure ulcers, device failures and patient falls.

ADVOCACY

Any activity done to help an individual or group get something they desire.

ADVOCATE

A person within the health care system who speaks for the patient and who makes certain that the patient receives the necessary services. This function is often performed by a case manager.

AFFORDABLE CARE ACT (ACA)

The legislation that includes a long list of health-related provisions that began taking effect in 2010. The key provisions are to extend coverage to millions of uninsured Americans, to implement measures that will lower health care costs and improve system efficiency, and to eliminate industry practices that include denial of healthcare coverage due to pre-existing conditions. Also called the Patient Protection and Affordable Care Act (PPACA)

AFTER SALE SERVICE

The services provided to the healthcare entity after the product has been delivered. This often includes repair, maintenance and/or telephone support.

AGAINST MEDICAL ADVICE (AMA)

A term used when a patient checks themselves out of a hospital or healthcare facility against the advice of a physician.

AGING

A medical billing term that refers to the length of time an invoice has been outstanding. It helps determine the financial health of the healthcare facility's customers, and therefore the health of their business or in the case of a patient their ability to pay.

AGREEMENT

A formal written document entered into at the end of the procurement process.

ALLERGY/IMMUNOLOGY

The diagnosis and treatment of allergic and immunologic diseases such as asthma or hay fever and drug and food allergies.

ALLIED HEALTH PROFESSIONAL (AHP)

An individual trained to support, complement, or supplement the professional functions of physicians, dentists, and other health professionals in the delivery of health care to patients. Such an individual is professionally educated and certified as a non-physician healthcare provider. Examples of AHPs include physician assistants, dental hygienists, medical technicians, nurse midwives, nurse practitioners, physical therapists, psychologists, and nurse anesthetists.

ALLOPATHIC

One of two schools of medicine that treat disease by using substances or techniques to oppose or suppress symptoms. The other school of medicine is osteopathic.

ALLOWABLE CHARGE

The maximum fee that a third party will reimburse a hospital or provider for a given service.

ALLOWABLE COST

Items or elements of a hospital's costs that are reimbursable under a payment formula. Allowable costs may exclude uncovered services, luxury items or accommodations, unreasonable or unnecessary costs and/or expenditures.

ALLOWANCE

The difference between gross revenue from services rendered and amounts received (or to be received) from patients or third-party payers.

ALL-PAYER SYSTEM

A plan requiring all payers of health care bills—the government, private insurers or an individual—to pay the same price for the same medical service. Uniform fees would eliminate cost shifting.

ALTERNATE

A substitute offer of goods and services which is at least a functional equal in features, performance and use and which materially does not deviate from one or more of the specifications in a competitive solicitation.

ALTERNATE CARE

Medical care received in lieu of inpatient hospitalization. Examples include outpatient surgery, home health care and skilled nursing facility care.

ALTERNATIVE BIRTHING CENTER

A room that is decorated in a homelike fashion and that is intended for a mother with a low risk pregnancy to use during labor and delivery.

ALTERNATIVE MEDICINE

Medical techniques that have traditionally been considered outside the boundaries of standard medical practice but are now eligible for coverage. Examples may include: Acupuncture, compounded medications, midwives, and osteopathic treatments.

AMBULATORY

Describes a patient capable of moving about from place to place and who is not confined to a bed.

AMBULATORY CARE (AC)

Health services that are provided on an outpatient basis. The services may be provided at a hospital or a free-standing facility. They may include diagnosis, observation, consultation, intervention, treatment or rehabilitation services.

AMBULATORY PAYMENT CLASSIFICATION (APC)

The method used by the Centers for Medicare & Medicaid Services (CMS) to implement prospective payment for ambulatory procedures. Many different ambulatory procedures are placed into groups for purposes of payment. They may include diagnosis, observation, consultation, intervention, treatment or rehabilitation services.

AMBULATORY SERVICES

Medical care that is provided on an outpatient basis as a non-emergency such as at a physician office, clinic or hospital. It includes diagnosis, observation, consultation, treatment and rehabilitation services.

AMBULATORY SURGERY

Surgery that does not require an over-night stay. Also called Out-Patient Surgery or Same-Day Surgery.

AMBULATORY SURGERY CENTER (ASC)

Outpatient, same-day surgical procedures provided in a hospital or freestanding ambulatory surgery center. Surgery that doesn't require an overnight hospital stay. It is also called outpatient surgery or same-day surgery.

AMENDMENT

For the purposes of a contract, shall mean an agreement between the parties to change the contract after it is fully signed by both parties.

AMERICANS WITH DISABILITIES ACT (ADA)

Federal legislation passed in 1990 prohibiting discrimination on the basis of disability in employment, public services and accommodations, and telecommunications.

AMOUNT CHARGED

The amount a doctor or hospital bills a patient.

AMOUNT NOT COVERED

The fees an insurance company does not pay. It includes deductibles, co-insurances and charges for non-covered services.

AMOUNT OF CONTRACT

The total financial obligation incurred by the hospital.

AMOUNT PAID

The monetary amount a patient pays for a doctor or hospital visit.

AMOUNT PAYABLE BY PLAN

The amount an insurer pays for patient treatment, minus any deductibles, coinsurance or charges for non-covered services.

AMORTIZATION

The write-off over a specified period of time of intangible assets.

ANCILLARY SERVICES

Services other than room, board, medical and nursing services provided to hospital or hospice patients during their stay. Examples are pharmacy, laboratory, radiology and therapy services.

ANESTHESIA

The use of drugs that cause a patient to lose sensation and go to sleep for a procedure (general anesthesia) or to numb an area for a procedure (local anesthesia). Another option is a block, which can keep an extremity numb for up to 36 hours. The type of anesthesia used depends on the patient's history, the procedure and other factors.

ANESTHETIC AGENT

The specific drug used to reduce or abolish the sensation of pain during anesthesia. Examples Include, e.g. halothane, enfluorane and isoflurane.

ANESTHESIOLOGY

Supervises and administers drugs and other agents to alleviate discomfort during operations and other medical procedures. Prior to surgery, an anesthesiologist meets with the patient to discuss anesthesia options and to answer questions. Anesthesia choices may vary, depending on the surgery being performed and the patient's health. General anesthesia keeps patients in a deep state of sleep, while regional anesthesia numbs the area around the surgery site. Throughout the procedure, the anesthesiologist monitors the patient's vital signs and responses. The anesthesiology staff also assists in planning post-operative pain management. After surgery, their help extends to patients moved to the Post Anesthesia Care Unit (PACU) and/or the Critical Care Unit. They strive to keep patients comfortable throughout and after their surgery experience.

ANGIOGRAPHY

The radiological examination of the blood vessels after injection of a dye opaque to X-rays.

ANGIOPLASTY

Plastic surgery of blood vessels. Often, a small balloon is inserted into a vein or artery and expanded to clear a blockage and calcified build-up on the lining of the vessel.

ANTERIOR

Before, in relation to time or space. The front surface of the body.

ANTIBIOTIC RESISTANCE

A broad term that encompasses resistance to many different types of pathogens such as bacteria, viruses and fungi.

ANTIBIOTICS

Drugs taken to prevent infections and kill bacteria.

ANTITRUST

A legal term that ensures that sellers do not attempt to restrain trade or fix their prices for goods and services in a market.

APGAR SCORE

An objective numerical summary of a newborn's condition at birth based on five different scores (heart rate, respiratory effort, muscle tone, skin color and response to a catheter in the nostril) measured at 1 minute and 5 minutes. Each of these receives a score of 0, 1 or 2. A score of 10 means the infant is in the best possible condition while a score of 3 means the infant needs to be resuscitated.

APNEA

An absence of breathing.

APPEAL

The process by which a patient, doctor, or hospital can disagree with the health plan's decision to not pay for care.

APPLIED TO DEDUCTIBLE

An amount that is subtracted from the insurance deductible amount, i.e., a credit towards the deductible payment.

APPROVAL LEVEL

The criteria, which is often monetary, that sets limits on the size and nature of business transactions that can be entered into by an individual based upon their role and level in the organization.

APPROVED VENDOR LIST

A list of all of the suppliers that are approved for doing business with the healthcare entity by procurement.

ARTERIAL LINE

A small hollow tube that is usually placed in an artery of the wrist, groin or ankle. It monitors blood pressure and allows nurses to draw blood for testing.

ARTHROSCOPY

Minimally invasive surgery on a joint.

ASSESSMENT

The evaluation of the health status of an individual that is done by performing a physical examination following a family history.

ASSET

Any owned physical equipment having economic value to the hospital.

ASSIGNMENT

An agreement a patient signs that allows an insurance company to pay a doctor or hospital directly.

ASSIGNMENT OF BENEFITS

A written authorization, signed by the patient or policyholder, to pay benefits directly to the hospital. It is usually acquired at the time of admission and imperative to be obtained prior to discharge. An assignment of benefits does not guarantee payment.

ATTENDING PHYSICIAN

The doctor who is responsible for the patient's care, usually in a hospital setting.

AUDIOLOGY

The services provided that relate to the hearing impaired and whose hearing cannot be improved by medical or surgical treatment. Specialist provide screening, evaluation and treatment programs.

AUTHORIZATION

This applies when a patient's health insurance plan requires them to get permission from their insurance provider before obtaining certain healthcare services. A patient may be denied insurance coverage if they see a healthcare provider for a service that needed authorization from their insurance company first.

AUTISM CENTER

Within a Children's hospital it is the center that provides assessment, diagnosis, treatment and support for autism spectrum disorders for babies, children and young adults.

AUTO RESUPPLY

The process of delivering a product directly to a department or nursing unit floor from the supply chain area without the user having to generate a requisition.

AUTHORIZATION NUMBER

A number stating that a patient's treatment has been approved by his or her insurance plan.

AUTONOMOUS DELIVERY ROBOT

A robot that performs behaviors or tasks with a high degree of independence from external control. Within hospitals these are being used to deliver linens, medical supplies or food to a unit.

AUXILIARY

A group of volunteers from the community that assist the hospital in carrying out its mission and who serves as a link between the hospital and the community.

AVAILABLE BEDS

The total number of beds within a healthcare facility that are maintained and staffed to provide health care.

AVERAGE AGE OF PLANT

The average age (in years) of buildings and equipment. The older the average age, the greater the short term need for capital resources. Many hospital also report a separate metric for the average age of their buildings and equipment separately.

AVERAGE COVERED CHARGES

The hospital's average charge for services covered by Medicare for all discharges in the diagnosis related group. These will vary from hospital to hospital because of differences in hospital charge structures.

AVERAGE DAILY CENSUS (ADC)

The average number of hospital inpatients per day over a given period that is calculated by dividing the total number of patient days during a given period by the number of calendar days in that period.

AVERAGE LENGTH OF STAY (ALOS)

The average number of days patients are in a hospital receiving inpatient care. It is calculated by dividing total patient days by the number of discharge days.

AVERAGE LIFE

The estimated useful-life expectancy of an asset subject to depreciation.

AVERAGE OR TURNOVER TIME

This Operating Room key performance indicator measures the average time elapsed between surgical cases. It is often defined as the time period from the prior patient exiting the OR to the following patient entering the OR. This includes clean-up and set-up time, but not delays between cases caused by a gap in the schedule.

AVERAGE PAYMENT PERIOD

A measure of how efficiently the hospital or healthcare facility pays its bills. It is measured in days.

AVERAGE WHOLESALER PRICE (AWP)

For brand-name pharmaceuticals, the Average Wholesale Price, as stated by the manufacturer is used as a basis for determining discounts and rebates.

AWARD

The acceptance of a bid or proposal; the presentation of a purchase agreement or contract to a bidder.

BACHELOR OF SCIENCE IN NURSING (BSN, BScN)

An academic degree in the science and principles of nursing, granted by an accredited tertiary education provider. In some countries it is a Bachelor of Nursing (BN) or Bachelor of Science (BS) with a Major in Nursing.

BACKORDERS

Information that sufficient quantities of an ordered item are not currently available. Usually a date or a number of days will be provided to tell the purchaser when the item(s) will be available.

BAD DEBT

Charges for care provided to patients who are financially able to pay but refuse to do so. It results when patients do not pay the bills for which payment was expected. It occurs for a variety of reasons, such as when uninsured patients have incomes above the guidelines for charity care, but still cannot afford the cost of their care.

BALANCE BILL

The amount doctors and hospitals charge a patient after their health plan, insurance company or Medicare has paid its approved amount.

BALANCE SHEET

A statement of assets and liabilities.

BALLOON PAYMENT

The final payment of a debt obligation which is always much larger than the preceding payments.

BAR CODE

A small image of lines (bars) and spaces that encodes information in a machine readable form that is used to identify materials coming into hospitals and those generated within a hospital, such as laboratory specimens, medical records, x-rays and drugs.

BARIATRIC PRODUCTS

Products that are designed to have a load bearing capacity of at least 300 and intended for patients with excessive body weight.

BARIATRIC SURGERY

Surgery of the stomach and/or intestines that helps an individual with extreme obesity lose weight. The weight loss is achieved by reducing the size of the stomach with a gastric band, through removal of a portion of the stomach or by resecting and re-routing the small intestine to a small stomach pouch which is called gastric bypass surgery.

BASSINET

A bed that is utilized for newborn infants. The number of bassinets is included in the number of available beds.

BED-SIZE

The total number of beds in a hospital that are maintained regularly for use during a reporting period.

BED TURN-OVER RATE

The number of times a hospital bed changes patients over a given period of time.

BEDS-AVAILABLE

The number of hospital beds which are regularly maintained and staffed and immediately available for the care of admitted patients.

BEDS-LICENSED

Number of beds that a hospital is licensed or certified by the state to maintain.

BEDS STAFFED

The number of beds a hospital actually operates.

BEHAVIORAL HEALTHCARE

The provision of mental health and chemical dependency (or substance abuse) services.

BENCHMARKING

A process which identifies best practices and performance standards (benchmarks) as a measurement and performance improvement mechanism. By comparing one hospital against a national or regional benchmark, hospitals are able to establish measurable goals as part of the Strategic Planning and Total Quality Management (TQM) processes.

BENEFICIARY

A person covered by health insurance and who receives benefits through that coverage.

BENEFICIARY ELIGIBILITY VERIFICATION

The means by which doctors and hospitals use to obtain information about whether a patient has insurance coverage.

BENEFICIARY LIABILITY

A statement that a patient is responsible for some portion of the charges.

BENEFIT

The amount an insurance company will pay for medical services.

BENEFIT MAXIMUM

The maximum payment amount that an insurance policy will pay for benefits.

BENEFIT PACKAGE

The list of covered services such as physician visits, hospitalizations, prescription drugs, that are covered by an insurance policy or health plan. The benefit package will specify any cost-sharing requirements for services, limits on particular services, and annual or lifetime spending limits.

BENEFIT PERIOD

The time period for which payments for benefits of an insurance policy are available.

BENIGN

Denoting the mild character of an illness or the nonmalignant character of an abnormal tissue growth.

BEST PRACTICES

The most up-to-date patient care practices that are believed to result in the best patient outcomes and to minimize a patients' risk of death or complications. Best practices may be identified using benchmarking, expert opinion, or scientific data.

BID

A written offer to perform a contract to purchase or supply goods and/or services in response to an Invitation to Bid (ITB), Request for Proposal (RFP) or other type of solicitation.

BID EVALUATION

The process of examining a bid after opening to determine the bidder's responsibility, responsiveness to requirements, and to ascertain other characteristics of the bid that relate to determination of the successful bidder.

BID LIST

List of potential bidders maintained by hospital procurement from which names may be drawn for solicitation of bids, quotes or proposals.

BID OPENING

The formal process through which bids are opened and the contents revealed for the first time.

BID SOLICITATION

The process of notifying potential bidders of an opportunity to bid on a project. Also called an invitation to bid, request of proposals, request for quotations, and a request for sealed bids.

BIDDER

A supplier who submits a bid, quotation or proposal.

BIDDERS CONFERENCE

A meeting chaired by hospital procurement to discuss with the potential bidder's the technical, operational and performance specifications and other issues related to the bid solicitation.

BIG DATA

Refers to large datasets that a company analyzes for patterns or trends.

BILIRUBIN

A yellow-orange pigment that is a normal waste product from the breakdown of hemoglobin from red blood cells. When bilirubin accumulates, it makes the skin and eyes look yellow, a condition called jaundice.

BILL

The printed summary of a medical bill. Also called a statement.

BILLING DEPARTMENT

The functional area responsible for computing the patient's hospital bill and sending an invoice to the insurance company and/or patient. It is also called accounts payable.

BILL OF LADING

A contract and document that contains the terms and conditions between the shipper and carrier.

BIN LOCATION

The location on a storage shelf where a supply item is placed until needed.

BIO-MEDICAL ENGINEERING DEPARTMENT

A hospital department that provides engineering services to the healthcare delivery system by assuring the safe and effective use of medical technology, improved patient outcomes and enhanced patient care in a cost effective manner.

BIOSIMILAR

A biological product that is approved based on showing that it is highly similar or an almost identical copy to an FDA-approved biological product whose patent has expired. It must have no clinically meaningful differences in terms of safety and effectiveness from the reference product.

BIOSTATISTICS

The branch of statistics dealing with data related to living organisms. Examples of numeric data on the general health of a population include births, deaths, incidence of disease, injuries etc.

BILLED CHARGES

The actual monetary amount billed by a physician or other healthcare service provider for a particular service.

BIOPSY

Removal of living tissue and then examination through a microscope to determine the precise nature of a pathological process.

BIRTHDAY RULE

Related to the coordination of benefits and determination of the primary payer when a child is covered by both parents' health insurance plans. This applies to non-divorced parents. The insurer of the parent whose birthday month falls first in the year is the primary payer.

BIRTHING ROOM/LABOR AND DELIVERY ROOM (LDR, LDRP)

Combines labor and delivery in a one room that has a homelike décor. An LDR room combines three phases: labor, delivery and recovery. In LDRP, four stages of the birth process are included: labor, delivery, recovery and postpartum.

BIRTH DEFECT

Any defect to a baby at birth.

BIRTHS

The total number of infants born in the hospital during the reporting period. Births do not include infants transferred from other institutions.

BLANKET PURCHASE ORDER

An order the healthcare entity makes with a supplier that contains multiple delivery dates scheduled over a period of time usually at predetermined prices.

BLOCK SCHEDULING

The practice by which a hospital or surgicenter assigns a specific operating room on a specific day(s) to a surgeon or surgical group.

BLOOD AND MARROW TRANSPLANTATION (BMT)

A treatment center with expertise in all areas of hematopoietic cell transplantation that offers a full complement of transplantation services such as donor evaluation, recipient evaluation, donor searches, stem cell collection, autologous transplants, sibling transplants, unrelated donor transplants and transplantation using bone marrow, cord blood, and peripheral blood stem cells and transplantation for both malignant (cancer) diseases and non-malignant diseases.

BLOOD BANK

Draws, processes, stores, and delivers blood to hospital departments.

BLOOD GAS

An arterial blood test used to evaluate a patient's level of oxygen, carbon dioxide and acid. This test is significant because it helps to evaluate respiratory status.

BLOOD UREA NITROGEN (BUN)

A blood test that measures the urea level of the blood. It describes how well the kidneys are functioning.

BLOODBORNE PATHOGENS (BBP)

Pathogenic microorganisms that are present in human blood and that can cause disease in humans. These pathogens include, but are not limited to, hepatitis B virus (HBV) and human immunodeficiency virus (HIV).

BOARD CERTIFICATION

The process by which physicians are certified within a specialty or a sub-specialty.

BOARD CERTIFIED

Board certified in medicine is the outcome of the process by which a medical credentialing organization (a Board) certifies that a health professional is competent to practice as a specialist in the designated field. The physician or other health professional must meet the requirements set by the Board for his or her specialty, such as working in the field for a certain period of time, performing a certain number procedures, and taking an examination.

BOARD-CERTIFIED SURGEON

A surgeon who has met the standards of excellence established and maintained by the American Board of Surgery (ABS).

BOARD DESIGNATED FUNDS

Unrestricted funds designated by the Governing Board for specific projects.

BOARD DESIGNATED INVESTMENT FUNDS

Unrestricted funds that have been designated to produce income, through prudent investment, by the Governing Board of the hospital.

BOARD ELIGIBLE

A physician who has completed the requirements for admission to a medical specialty board examination but has not taken and passed the examination.

BOARD OF COMMISSIONERS

The governing body of the Joint Commission that provides policy leadership and oversight.

BOARD OF TRUSTEES

The legal entity ultimately responsible for hospital policy, organization, management, and quality of care. Also called the governing board, commissioners, or directors. It is called a Board of Trustees in a For-Profit hospital. They are accountable to the owner(s) of the hospital, which is a corporation.

BOND DISCOUNT

The excess of the face amount of a bond (or class of bonds) over the net amount yielded from its sale.

BOND PREMIUM

The net amount yielded by the sale of a bond (or class of bonds) in excess of its face value.

BONDS

A written certificate of indebtedness that is binding to one or more parties as surety for another.

BRADYCARDIA

A slow heart rate, usually below 60 beats per minute.

BRAIN DEATH

Total irreversible cessation of cerebral function along with spontaneous function of the circulatory and respiratory systems.

BRAIN SCAN

A diagnostic test using computerized axial tomography, magnetic resonance imaging or positron emission tomography to image the brain.

BRAND NAME DRUG

Prescription drugs that are marketed with a specific brand name by the company that manufactures it. Usually it's the same company that developed and patented it.

BREACH

The illegal access of a healthcare organization's information.

BREECH BIRTH

A birth whereby the infant emerges feet, buttocks or knees first.

BRONCHOSCOPY

A procedure that uses a flexible tube (called a bronchoscope) containing a fiber-optic cable that transmits images of the main airways of the lungs (the bronchi). This procedure helps to evaluate and diagnose lung problems or blockages, obtain samples of tissue and/or fluid, and/or to help remove a foreign body.

BUDGET

A statement that shows the units of service, revenue and operating expenses over a defined time period.

BUNDLED PAYMENT

A single, fixed payment whereby patients or insurers are charged one overall price for all services associated with a patient's condition and treatments over an episode of care. Hospitals and participating providers also receive one payment for the entire episode of care.

BUDGET YEAR (BY)

Fiscal period (usually 12 months) for anticipated expenses and revenues.

BURN CARE UNIT

Specialized care for severely burned patients in a distinct unit by specially trained personnel. This can consist of treatment of fresh burns and plastic reconstructive or restorative surgery as a result of a healed burn.

BUSINESS CASE

A detailed document that presents information on product, service, solution or other topic in order to make an informed business decision. It should include statistics and financial information.

BUSINESS OFFICE

The department responsible for the day-to-day business procedures which deal primarily with patient accounts (posting, billing and collections), accounts payable and payroll.

BUYING CENTER

A group of stakeholders that collaborate to make a decision on the purchase of a new product. Within a hospital setting this may be a value analysis committee, new product committee, technical evaluation committee or others.

BUYING GREEN

A product or service that reduces the impact on human health or the environment when compared with competitive products or services. Examples are those that contain recycled materials, minimize waste, conserve energy or water, and reduce the amount of toxics either disposed of or consumed.

BUYING TEAM

A group of individuals that offer ideas, arguments, agreement and a forum to discuss the full complement of needs for a product or a service. Within a hospital this is generally done within a committee structure.

CAFETERIA

The area of the hospital that provides food services for the medical staff, hospital inpatients, employees and visitors.

CAFETERIA BENEFIT PLAN

A plan that allows employees to pick and choose their benefit structure to meet their needs and requirements.

CANCER

A disease which involves malignant tumors capable of spreading. These can be systemic, such as leukemia, or organ specific, such as breast, kidney or lung cancer.

CAPITAL ASSET

Depreciable property of a fixed or permanent nature (e.g. buildings and equipment) that is not for sale in the regular course of business.

CAPITAL BUDGET

The part of the budget typically comprised of items that cost more than a fixed threshold (e.g.an expense >$5,000) and that has a useful life greater than 5 years.

CAPITAL COSTS

Expenditures for land, facilities, and major equipment.

CAPITAL EXPENDITURE

Any expenditure for the acquisition, replacement, modernization, or expansion of a facility or equipment which is not properly chargeable as an expense for operation and maintenance. Example: new buildings or equipment with a useful life of several years.

CAPITAL EXPENSE

Costs for a physical improvement or a piece of equipment that will provide benefit over a number of years. Capital expenses are typically significant in monetary size and scope.

CAPITAL LEASE

A lease which meets one of the following four criteria:

- The present value of the minimum lease payments is 90 percent or more of the fair value of the property to the lessor.

- The lease term is 75 percent or more of the leased property's estimated economic life.

- The lease contains a bargain (less than fair value) purchased option.

- Ownership is transferred to the lessee by the end of the lease terms.

CAPITALIZE

Recording of an expenditure as an asset providing a future benefit as opposed to an expense during the period of its purchase.

CAPITATION

When the provider is paid a fixed dollar amount per month for each of the patients for whom he/she agrees to provide care, regardless of whether those patients seek care or not.

CARE CONTINUUM

The range of health services and coordination to a patient to address his or her health and wellness needs over time. This includes inpatient, outpatient, in home, rehabilitation, nursing, and remote monitoring.

CARDIAC CARE UNIT (CCU)

An adult critical care unit providing comprehensive care for critically ill patients with a primary cardiac diagnosis. The unit is staffed with specially trained personnel that offers more intensive, focused cardiac care than general medical and surgical care. Also called a Cardiac Intensive Care Unit (CICU) in some facilities.

CARDIAC CATHETERIZATION

The passage of a flexible surgical instrument through a vein in the arm, leg or neck and then into the heart to obtain blood samples or perform other tests.

CARDIAC CATHETERIZATION LABORATORY

The functional area that provides special diagnostic procedures for cardiac patients.

CARDIAC ELECTROPHYSIOLOGY

A branch of cardiology that deals with the diagnosis and treatment of heart rhythm disorders. These physicians perform ablation and implant and manage cardiac devices. After the standard cardiology fellowship they typically study an extra year (or two).

CARDIAC INTENSIVE CARE UNIT (CICU)

An adult critical care unit providing comprehensive care for critically ill patients with a primary cardiac diagnosis. The unit is staffed with specially trained personnel that offers more intensive, focused cardiac care than general medical and surgical care. Also called a Cardiac Care Unit (CCU) in some facilities.

CARDIAC STRESS TEST

A recording of the heart's activity while a patient is exercising. Their heart is monitored by using electrodes to record the electrical activity it makes while simultaneously seeing how the blood pressure and pulse change over the course of the test.

CARDIOLOGY

The area of medicine that specializes in the diagnosis, treatment and prevention of heart disease.

CARDIOLOGY CLINIC

Out-patient services provided in a clinic for the study of the heart.

CARDIOPULMONARY BYPASS (CPB)

Use of a machine that takes over the function of the heart and lungs during heart surgery by circulating the blood returning to the heart through a machine instead. This technology allows surgery to be performed on a non-beating heart.

CARDIO-PULMONARY CARE DEPARTMENT

The department that employs licensed respiratory therapists that are trained to assess, treat, manage, control, educate and care for patients with cardiopulmonary problems. Most departments conduct EKGs, cardiac stress tests, EEG tests, pulmonary function testing, Holter and event monitoring, provide adult and pediatric respiratory care, and testing of oxygen levels for patients admitted to the hospital and on an outpatient basis. Also called Respiratory Care Department.

CARDIO-PULMONARY RESUSCITATION (CPR)

An emergency lifesaving procedure that is done when someone's breathing or heartbeat has stopped. This can happen after an electric shock, heart attack, or drowning.

CARDIOVASCULAR SURGERY

Surgeons who have extensive training in cardiovascular and thoracic physiology and disease processes. They perform numerous procedures, including specialty operative procedures such as coronary artery bypass, valvular heart disease repair and aortic and mitral valve replacement.

C-ARM

A mobile fluoroscopy system used for studies ranging from orthopedics to cardiology.

CARE CONTINUUM

The range of health services and coordination to a patient to address his or her health and wellness needs over time. This includes inpatient, outpatient, in home, rehabilitation, nursing, and remote monitoring.

CAREGIVER

Someone who gives care to another person. There are two types of caregivers: medical caregivers and non-medical caregivers. Medical caregivers, such as registered nurses, provide care to patients with medical requirements. Non-medical caregivers, such as home health aides, help individuals with activities of daily living (ADLs) and companionship.

CARE GUIDELINES

A set of medical treatments for a particular condition or group of patients that has been reviewed and endorsed by a national organization.

CARE PLAN

A plan-of-care developed from the assessment of the patient and his/her diagnosis.

CARRIER

The insurance company or HMO offering a health plan.

CARVE OUT

Within health insurance it is when the employer does not pay for certain services such as vison services etc.

CASE CART

A handcart that contains all of the supplies required to perform a procedure for a specific surgical case.

CASE DURATION

This Operating Room key performance indicator can be measured differently by each facility. Some examples include:

- From the time the patient is in the surgical suite to when the patient is out of the room.

- The time from the start of the OR room set-up (before the case) to the completion of room clean-up (after the case).

- Cut (incision) to close time.

CASE DURATION ACCURACY

This Operating Room key performance indicator measures the percentage of OR cases with durations that are accurately estimated. Typically, an accurate estimate is when the variance between the actual and scheduled case duration is within 15 minutes.

CASE HISTORY

This is a patient's complete medical record and includes immunizations, allergies, hospitalizations, therapies etc.

CASE MANAGEMENT

A collaborative process that assesses, plans, implements, evaluates, and coordinates options and services to ensure cost-effective patient outcomes in the most cost effective manner.

CASE MANAGEMENT DEPARTMENT

The department that provides patient case assessment, treatment planning, referral, and follow-up. Usually it is affiliated with or part of the Social Services Department.

CASE MINUTES

Reflects the total number of minutes of surgery each month. When this metric is compared to volume it helps to show growth patterns. For example: a small increase in case volumes with a large increase in minutes should mean that surgeons are preforming longer more complex surgeries. If there is a small increase in case volume and a small increase in minutes, then it probably means shorter surgical cases are being performed.

CASE MIX

Categories of patients classified by disease, procedure, method of payment, or other characteristics in an institution at a given time, usually measured by counting or aggregating groups of patients sharing one or more characteristics.

CASE MIX INDEX (CMI)

An indicator of the level of diversity and clinical complexity of the patients treated by a provider and its costliness. A hospital's CMI represents the average diagnosis-related group (DRG) relative weight for that hospital. It is calculated by summing the DRG weights for all Medicare discharges and dividing by the number of discharges. CMIs are calculated using both transfer-adjusted cases and unadjusted cases. The higher the CMI is, the sicker its patients, and the more resources that patients will require during treatment.

CASE VOLUME

This Operating Room key performance indicator reflects the total number of surgical cases over a defined time period. It is typically measured for both in-patient and out-patient surgeries. While it is tracked monthly the best measure is the average number of cases per OR per year because this measurement takes into account surgeon vacations and attendance at medical conventions.

CATCHMENT AREA

Geographic area defined and served by a hospital on the basis of such factors as population distribution, natural geographic boundaries and transportation accessibility.

CATEGORY MANAGEMENT

Involves grouping related products or services together so that "pools of spend "are managed in a more precise manner to cut overall spend.

CENSUS

Average number of inpatients, excluding newborns, receiving care each day as of midnight in a facility.

CENTERS FOR MEDICARE AND MEDICAID SERVICES (CMS)

An agency within the US Department of Health & Human Services responsible for administration of several key federal health care programs. They are responsible for managing Medicare (the federal health insurance program for seniors) and Medicaid (the federal needs-based program). CMS also runs the State Children's Health Insurance Program (SCHIP), which is jointly financed by the Federal and State governments and administered by individual States.

CENTERS OF EXCELLENCE

Hospitals with staffing and equipment that specialize in difficult, complex, and expensive tertiary care procedures, such as heart, kidney or other organ transplants or coronary artery bypass surgery.

CENTRAL SERVICE

The service area within the hospital in which medical and surgical supplies and equipment (both sterile and non-sterile) are cleaned, processed, stored and issued for patient care. The primary customer of Central Services is the Operating Room. This department is also called the Sterile Processing Department.

CERTIFICATE OF BID OPENING

A certification by the person conducting a bid that the opening of all timely proposals received was held at the specified time and place.

CERTIFICATE OF INSURANCE

A printed description that defines in writing the benefits and coverage provisions forming the contract between the carrier and the customer. It defines what is covered, what is not and the dollar limits.

CERTIFICATE OF NEED (CON)

A document, provided by a state governing board to a healthcare institution (at the institution's request) which allows the institution to build additional physical facilities and/or add equipment or new services. Some states require a CON while others do not.

CERTIFICATION

The formal process by which an authorized governmental or non-governmental organization evaluates and recognizes either an individual or an organization as meeting pre-determined requirements or criteria.

CHAMPUS

The health plan for the dependents of active duty military personnel and retired military personnel and their dependents. CHAMPUS stands for Civilian Health and Medical Program for the Uniformed Services.

CHANGE ORDER

Formal notification that a purchase order must be modified in some way.

CHAPLAINCY/PASTORAL CARE SERVICES

Spirituality and faith are an important part of health and recovery. Hospital chaplains are professionally trained to offer patient-centered care through pre-op and post-op visits, crisis counseling, chronic and rehabilitation support service, care for persons facing death, and bereavement care. A hospital chapel is also often available.

CHARGE

The price a healthcare provider indicates it is owed for a service. This is not necessarily what it expects to receive.

CHARGE MASTER

A list of all tests, orders, or procedures performed by the hospital and billable to the patient or the patient's health insurance provider.

CHARGE NURSE

A registered nurse assigned to be in charge of a hospital nursing unit.

CHARGEABLE SUPPLIES

Supplies that may be charged to a patient's bill for care provided.

CHARGE CAPTURE

The digital capture of information for billable services for use in a medical claim document.

CHARGES

The amount billed by a hospital for services provided. A charge generally includes the cost plus an operating margin. Many payers pay a discounted rate, negotiated rate or government set rate.

CHARITY CARE

The difference between full-established charges for services rendered to patients who are not able to pay for all or part of the services provided and the amount paid by or on behalf of the patient, if any. Eligibility is sometimes determined from a sliding scale based on a percentage of the patient's income above the federal poverty level.

CHART OF ACCOUNTS

A list of accounts giving account names and numbers.

CHEMICAL DEPENDENCY SERVICES

Services and supplies used in the diagnosis and treatment of alcoholism, chemical dependency, and drug dependencies. These are defined and classified by the U.S. Department of Health and Human Services.

CHILDREN'S HEALTH INSURANCE PROGRAM (CHIP)

A state-administered program funded partly by the federal government that allows states to expand health coverage to uninsured, low-income children not eligible for Medicaid.

CHILDREN'S HOSPITAL

A hospital with a majority of its inpatients under the age of 18, which participates and is paid in the Medicare program as a Children's Hospital.

CHRONIC CARE

Treatment that is provided to people whose health problems are long-term and continuing.

CHRONIC ILLNESS

Diseases which are permanent, exhibit disability, are caused by nonreversible pathological alteration, require special training of the patient for rehabilitation, or may be expected to require a long period of supervision, observation, or care.

CHURCH OPERATED

Hospitals operated by a not-for-profit religious organization.

CLAIM

A bill for health services. Claims are sent by physicians and other providers, hospitals, laboratories, pharmacies, etc. to payers and patients for services rendered.

CLAIM NUMBER

A number assigned to a medical service.

CLAIMS MANAGEMENT

The process of managing healthcare claims from patients.

CLEAN CLAIM

A medical claim filed with a health insurance company that is free of errors and processed in a timely manner.

CLEARINGHOUSE

Facilities that review and correct medical claims as required before sending them to an insurance company for final processing.

CLINIC

This term can be defined in a number of ways. It may be a physician office, a facility for the diagnosis and treatment of outpatients or where graduate or under-graduate medical education is performed.

CLINIC VISITS

A visit by a patient to an outpatient facility for examination, diagnosis or treatment.

CLINICAL ASSESSMENT

An evaluation of a patient's physical condition and prognosis based on their medical history, laboratory results and physical examination.

CLINICAL DECISION SOFTWARE

An evidence-based computer program that helps providers make clinical decisions for their patients.

CLINICAL DEPARTMENT

In a departmentalized hospital, the medical staff organization is subdivided into major divisions such as medicine, surgery, obstetrics-gynecology, pediatrics and family medicine. Each clinical department has a chief or chairman and is responsible for setting and monitoring standards of professional and personal conduct of physicians within those departments.

CLINICAL HOURS PER CASE

Measures how much time the clinical staff (nurses, per-op and post-op staff and clinical support staff is spending with each patient.

CLINICAL INFORMATION SYSTEM

The software program that manages a hospital's administrative, medical, financial, and legal information services. The software stores, organizes, and supports data retrieval to improve efficiency and cost-effectiveness.

CLINICAL INTELLIGENCE

The knowledge and information resulting from the collection of clinical data to provide insights into how to deliver healthcare at higher quality and lower cost.

CLINICAL LABORATORY

The laboratory where blood, urine, and other tests are performed.

CLINICAL LABORATORY IMPROVEMENT AMENDMENT OF 1988 (CLIA 88)

A certification standard for laboratories. They were established to consolidate the requirements for Medicare participation with rules for laboratories engaged in interstate testing under the CLIA '67 program. The standards contain quality control and quality assurance, proficiency testing and personnel requirements.

CLINICAL MEASURES

Measures of therapeutic processes and patient outcomes that are assumed to represent the quality of care. Such metrics are tracked in order to determine performance in a given clinical area, such as heart attack, pneumonia, or hip and knee replacement.

CLINICAL PATHWAY

A patient care management tool that organizes, sequences, and times the major interventions of nursing staff, physicians, and other clinical departments for a particular clinical situation.

CLINICAL PERFORMANCE

The degree to which desired health objectives are accomplished by a clinician or healthcare organization.

CLINICAL PERFORMANCE MEASURE

A means for assessing the degree to which a provider competently and safely delivers clinical services that are appropriate for the patient in the desired time period.

CLINICAL PRACTICE GUIDELINES

A set of statements, directions, or principles presenting current or future rules or policy. Guidelines are usually based on scientific evidence, to assist clinicians in making appropriate healthcare decisions for specific clinical circumstances.

CLINICAL PRIVILEGES

The right to provide medical or surgical care services in the hospital, within well-defined limits, according to an individual's professional license, education, training, experience and current clinical competence. Hospital privileges must be delineated individually for each practitioner by the hospital board, based on medical staff recommendations. Also called Privileges, Staff Privileges or Medical Staff Privileges.

CLINICAL PSYCHOLOGY

The science of working with mental processes both normal and abnormal and their effects on human behavior.

CLINICAL RESEARCH

The science devoted to finding information that improves people's health by examining the safety and effectiveness of drugs, medical devices, diagnostic tests, and treatment intended for human use.

CLINICAL STATUS

A type of outcome measure that relates to an improvement in the biological health status of the patient.

CLINICAL TRIAL

A scientifically designed research study involving humans that is overseen by the FDA and that compares the effect of drugs, medical devices, diagnostic tests, and treatments.

CLINICIAN

A healthcare professional that uses direct observation and treatment of a patient. Examples are nurses, respiratory, speech, occupational and physical therapy.

CLOSE CALL

An event or situation that did not produce patient injury but could have, only because of chance. Also referred to as a "near miss."

COBRA

COBRA stands for the Consolidated Omnibus Budget Reconciliation Act of 1986. It is a temporary continuation of health care coverage at group rates that is available to certain former employees, retirees, spouses, and dependent children when coverage is lost due to a qualifying event, often as a loss of employment. Usually, COBRA participants pay the entire premium themselves.

CODE BLACK

This is a slang term that means a patient is having a cardiopulmonary arrest within a hospital or clinic that requires a team of clinicians (often called a "code team") to hurry to the designated location and begin immediate resuscitation. Each hospital decides how to handle the various types of emergencies. Some have specific code designations for cardiopulmonary arrests, bomb threats, child abductions or mass causalities. Colors, numbers or other designations can follow a "code' to provide specificity. Also called Code Blue or Code Red in some institutions.

CODE BLUE

This is a slang term that means a patient is having a cardiopulmonary arrest within a hospital or clinic that requires a team of clinicians (often called a "code team") to hurry to the designated location and begin immediate resuscitation. Each hospital decides how to handle the various types of emergencies. Some have specific code designations for cardiopulmonary arrests, bomb threats, child abductions or mass causalities. Colors, numbers or other designations can follow a "code' to provide specificity. Also called Code Black or Code Red in some institutions.

CODE RED

This is a slang term that means a patient is having a cardiopulmonary arrest within a hospital or clinic that requires a team of clinicians (often called a "code team") to hurry to the designated location and begin immediate resuscitation. Each hospital decides how to handle the various types of emergencies. Some have specific code designations for cardiopulmonary arrests, bomb threats, child abductions or mass causalities. Colors, numbers or other designations can follow a "code' to provide specificity. Also called Code Blue or Code Black in some institutions.

CODING

The process of translating a physician's documentation about a patient's medical condition and health services rendered into special medical codes that are then inserted into a claim for processing with an insurance company.

COGNITIVE BEHAVIORAL THERAPY (CBT)

A type of counseling that focuses on changing specific thoughts and patterns of behavior. It is often used to treat stress, depression, anxiety, panic disorders and chronic pain.

COHORT STUDY

A clinical research study in which people who presently have a certain condition or receive a particular treatment are followed over time and compared with another group of people who are not affected by the condition.

COINSURANCE

The cost-sharing portion of a bill that a patient must pay. It is calculated as a percent of the total bill.

COLLECTIONS

The department responsible for obtaining prompt payment from the patient or payer for services rendered.

COLON & RECTAL SURGERY

Surgery of the large intestine, rectum and related structures.

COLONOSCOPE

A flexible tube containing a fiber-optic cable with a light and camera at the end that is inserted through the rectum to view the inside of the colon.

COLONOSCOPY

A procedure whereby a physician uses a colonoscope to look into the rectum and colon.

CO-MORBID CONDITION

A medical condition that, along with the principal diagnosis, exists at admission and is expected to increase hospital length of stay by at least one day for most patients.

CO-MORBIDITY

Conditions that exist at the same time as the primary condition in a patient. For example many patients with chronic obstructive pulmonary disease (COPD) also have sleep apnea.

COMMUNITY HEALTH CENTERS

These are federally qualified health clinics that provide primary care services to patients regardless of their income or insurance status. Under federal law the health centers must be located in or targeted to serve medically underserved communities and offer a sliding fee scale based on a patient's ability to pay for care for the services rendered. They must also have community boards.

COMMUNITY HOSPITAL

All nonfederal, short-term general and specialty hospitals whose facilities and services are available to the public. (Specialty hospitals include long term acute care, rehabilitation, children's, heart or spine.) Another name for a licensed hospital that provides medical and nursing care for medical and surgical conditions. These institutions are located in both urban and rural areas.

COMPANION

Within the homecare environment it is someone that serves a non-medical role in a patient's life. Companion Care Services typically caters to seniors and they perform duties such as reminder services (medications, dates, routines), assisting with mobility, providing companionship, preparing meals and feeding, escorting to appointments, organizing and reading mail, entertaining etc.

COMPARATIVE EFFECTIVENESS RESEARCH (CER)

Research that is designed to influence healthcare decisions by providing evidence on the effectiveness, benefits, and harms of different treatment options. The evidence is generated from unbiased and well-constructed research studies that compare drugs, medical devices, tests, surgeries, and/or ways to deliver health care.

COMPETITION

The process by which vendors vie to secure the business of a purchaser by offering favorable terms such as price, quality, delivery and/or service.

COMPETITIVE BENCHMARKING

The process used to compare and rate a company's products or services against those of its competitors.

COMPETITIVE PROCUREMENT

The formal procedures developed by the hospital or health system that outlines the procurement and bid process. The intent is to show their process to be fair and impartial.

COMPETITIVE SOLICITATION

A generic term for a request for solicitation. The solicitation method used will be determined by the dollar amount of the requested item and the complexity of the project/product. Different types of solicitations include Request for Quote (RFQ), Request for Proposal (RFP), Invitation to Bid (ITB) and Request for Information (RFI).

COMPLETE BLOOD COUNT (CBC)

A blood test that is used to evaluate the overall health of an individual. It measures Red blood cells, which carry oxygen; White blood cells, which fight infection; Hemoglobin, the oxygen-carrying protein in red blood cells; Hematocrit, the proportion of red blood cells to the fluid component, or plasma, in the blood and Platelets, which help with blood clotting.

COMPLIANCE

A hospital program that provides regulatory oversight and education to ensure legal and ethical standards of conduct. It is used to reduce the potential for fraud and abuse in coding and billing.

COMPLICATION

A medical condition that arises during a course of inpatient hospital treatment and is expected to increase the length of stay by at least one day for most patients.

COMPLICATION RATE

The incidence of medical problems associated with a particular procedure or illness.

COMPOUNDED DRUG

A drug that is made by mixing ingredients (prescription and/or over-the-counter) together to mix a formulation that's not readily available or approved by the Food and Drug Administration, to meet a particular patient's requirements.

COMPREHENSIVE OUTPATIENT REHABILITATION FACILITY (CORF)

An outpatient facility that provides individuals with diagnostic, therapeutic and restorative services for rehabilitation. These services are only available under a doctor's order. Also commonly called an Outpatient Rehabilitation Center.

COMPRESSION STOCKINGS

Long tight socks that are worn after an operation to put pressure on the leg muscles, to avoid the formation of a blood clot.

COMPUTERIZED AXIAL TOMOGRAPHY (CAT)

Diagnostic equipment that produces cross-sectional images of the head and/or body.

COMPUTER PHYSICIAN ORDER ENTRY (CPOE)

An electronic prescribing system whereby physicians enter orders into a computer rather than on paper. The orders are then integrated with patient information, including laboratory and prescription data. The order is also automatically checked for potential errors or problems.

CONCURRENT REVIEW

The process in which a health care provider uses a screening method to review a procedure or hospital admission performed by a colleague to assess its necessity.

CONCURRENT SURGERIES

The practice whereby a surgeon splits his time between the operating room they are currently in and another where they were operating on a second patient at the same time. This is often a common practice in teaching hospitals.

CONFIDENTIALITY AGREEMENT

A legal agreement between two or more parties that signifies a confidential relationship exists between the parties. It's used when various entities or people become privy to sensitive corporate information, which should not be made available to the general public or to various competitors.

CONFLICT OF INTEREST

A situation where the personal interests of a contractor, public official or employee are, or appear to be, at odds with the best interests of the hospital.

CONGESTED HEART FAILURE (CHF)

When the heart cannot pump enough blood to meet the body's needs.

CONSCIOUS SEDATION

The use of sedatives and pain medicine during surgery in which the patient stays awake but probably will not remember the procedure.

CONSENT (FOR TREATMENT)

A written agreement signed by a patient that gives permission to receive medical services or treatment from doctors or hospitals.

CONSIGNMENT

The process whereby a supplier places products at the hospital location at no charge and does not receive payment until the items are used.

CONSULTATION

A discussion with another health care professional to obtain additional feedback during a patient diagnosis or treatment.

CONSUMERISM

A movement whereby consumers shop for healthcare and become more involved in their own health care decisions.

Continuing Medical Education (CME)

A process of ongoing education on the part of individual physicians and other medical professionals, who often in the context of professional requirements in specialty fields take courses, read medical journals, attend teaching programs and take self-study courses to keep up with medical improvements, procedures, drugs, etc.

Continuous Replenishment Process

A method used in inventory management that matches replenishment to actual usage. As supplies are used they are immediately replenished.

Continuous Quality Improvement (CQI)

A management approach to improving and maintaining quality that emphasizes internally driven and relatively continuous assessments of potential causes of quality defects, followed by action aimed either at avoiding a decrease in quality or else correcting it an early stage. Scientific methods are used to continually improve at work processes, and to empower all employees to engage in continuous improvement of their work.

Continuum of Care

The provision of coordinated healthcare services that encompass preventive care, primary care, acute care, chronic care, rehabilitative care and supportive care so as to maximize the value of services received by patients by providing continuity of care. The continuum of care focuses on prevention and early intervention for those who have been identified as high risk and provides easy transition from service to service as patient needs change.

Contract

All types of agreements, regardless of what they may be called, for the procurement of goods and services. A purchase order is a contract.

Contract Administrative Fee (CAF)

A fee paid by a manufacturer to a GPO, on behalf of the hospital member, for obtaining access to its members and doing business.

Contracting

The last stage in the process of sourcing strategically. It often includes issuing an RFP and/or negotiating with existing supplier(s) and then finalizing contractual terms and conditions.

Contract Management

Planned, ongoing or periodic activity that measures and ensures contractor compliance with the terms, conditions, requirements of a contract, and oftentimes the auditing of invoices.

CONTRACTED RATE

The price that an insurer and healthcare provider have agreed upon for payment for a specific service.

CONTRACTOR

A vendor from whom the hospital obtains commodities, services or technology. Also called a supplier or vendor.

CONTRACTUAL ADJUSTMENT

Bookkeeping adjustment to reflect uncollectible differences between established charges for services rendered to insured individuals and rates payable for those services under contracts with third party payers.

CONTRACTUAL ALLOWANCE

Negotiated discounts from hospital-established charges.

CONTRACT SERVICE

Services performed by an organization outside the hospital under the terms and conditions of a contract.

CONTRAINDICATION

A situation that will cause the administration of a drug or treatment to be harmful to an individual.

CONTROLLED DELIVERY MEDICINES

Medications that are slowly released into the body to reduce how fast the body absorbs the medicine. Also called extended release, modified-release, prolonged release, controlled-release, controlled delivery, slow release and sustained-release medicines.

CONTROLLED RELEASE MEDICINES

Medications that are slowly released into the body to reduce how fast the body absorbs the medicine. Also called extended release, modified-release, prolonged release, controlled delivery, slow release and sustained-release medicines.

COORDINATION OF BENEFITS (COB)

A method to determine which insurance company is responsible for payment when a patient has more than one insurance plan. Oftentimes, an individual can have more than one kind of insurance coverage. For example: one plan from their employer and one from their spouse's employer. In that case, the two health plans work together to coordinate which one pays first, and how much. This process is called coordination of benefits.

COORDINATION OF CARE

The systems and procedures that ensure the patient and clinicians have access to, and take into consideration, all of the required information on the patient's condition and treatment (actual and potential) to ensure that the patient receives appropriate healthcare services.

CO-PAYMENT (CO-PAY)

A cost-sharing arrangement in which an insured person pays a specified charge for a specific service, such as $10 for a physician office visit. The insured is usually responsible for payment at the time the health care is rendered. Typical co-payments are fixed or variable flat amounts for physician office visits, prescriptions, or hospital services.

CORE COMPETENCIES

The combination of knowledge and technical ability that allows a hospital to be competitive in the local market.

CORE MEASURES

A set of care processes which were developed by The Joint Commission to improve the quality of health care by implementing a national, standardized performance measurement system. The Core Measures were derived largely from a set of quality indicators defined by the Centers for Medicare and Medicaid Services (CMS). They have been shown to reduce the risk of complications, prevent recurrences and otherwise treat the majority of patients who come to a hospital for treatment of a condition or illness. Core Measures help hospitals improve the quality of patient care by focusing on the actual results of care.

COST ACCOUNTING

An accounting system arriving at charges by hospitals or healthcare providers based on actual costs for services rendered.

COST ADJUSTMENT

The monetary difference between the charge and the contracted rate.

COST ALLOCATION

The apportionment of the costs of nonrevenue producing cost centers to revenue producing centers.

COST AVOIDANCE

The dollar amount averted by not bringing in a new product into the healthcare organization.

COST-BASED REIMBURSEMENT

When a third party pays the hospital for the care received by covered patients at cost.

COST-BENEFIT ANALYSIS

An analytical approach that compares the financial costs to the benefits in a defined period of time to assist in determining which products or projects should be funded.

COST CENTER

A division, department, service, or unit performing functional activities within a hospital. In each area, revenues and expenses are tracked.

COST CONTAINMENT

Control or reduction of inefficiencies in the consumption, allocation or production of hospital products and services that contribute to higher-than-necessary costs.

COST CONTROL

The process that hospitals and other healthcare facilities use to monitor and regulate expenses.

COST EFFECTIVENESS ANALYSIS

A type of analysis that is used when the benefits cannot be measured in monetary terms.

COST-RELATED REIMBURSEMENT

Method of payment for healthcare services in which the insurer pays the hospital based on the hospital's cost of delivering care.

COST REPORT

The report Medicare requires from providers on an annual basis to a Medicare Administrative Contractor (MAC) in order to make a proper determination of amounts payable. The cost report contains provider information such as facility characteristics, utilization data, cost and charges by cost center (in total and for Medicare), Medicare settlement data, and financial statement data.

COST SHARING

The portion of health expenses that a health plans beneficiary must pay including deductibles, co-payments and coinsurance.

COST-TO-CHARGE RATIO

A cost-finding measure derived from applying the ratio of third party charges to total charges against the total operating costs in a hospital operating department.

COST VARIANCE

A term used in cost accounting that describes the differences between actual costs and what was budgeted or expected.

COVERED BENEFIT

A health service or item that is included in a health plan and that is paid either partially or fully.

COVERED CHARGES

The charges for which an insurance provider will consider payment.

COVERED DAYS

The number of days that an insurance provider pays for in full or in part.

COVERED SERVICES AND SUPPLIES

A description of the services and supplies that are covered and reimbursable under a healthcare plan.

CPT CODE

The code used to identify procedures performed; required by most insurance companies. CPT (Current Procedures Terminology) is developed and approved by the American Medical Association.

CREDENTIALING AND PRIVILEGING

Process by which hospitals and health facilities determine the scope of practice of practitioners providing services in the hospital. The criteria for granting privileges or credentialing are determined by the hospital and include checking a practitioner's references and documenting his/her credentials, which includes training and education, experience, demonstrated ability, licensure verification and malpractice insurance. The hospital governing board has ultimate accountability for physician credentialing but usually delegates the process to the medical staff committee.

CRITERIA

The expected levels of achievement against which performance or quality may be compared.

CRITICAL ACCESS HOSPITAL (CAH)

A rural hospital that meets federally mandated criteria that enables the hospital to receive cost-based reimbursement for Medicare services.

CRITICAL CARE MEDICINE

The specialized care of patients with life-threatening conditions, such as a coma, trauma, heart failure, organ failure and respiratory conditions.

CRITICAL CARE NURSE

A licensed professional nurse who is responsible for ensuring that acutely and critically ill patients receive optimal care.

CRITICAL CARE NURSING

A specialty within nursing that focuses on human responses to life-threatening problems.

CRITICAL CARE UNIT (CCU)

Also called intensive care. This is the highest level of care for seriously ill patients. Optional specialty designations include burn care, cardio-thoracic, coronary care, medical, neurology, pulmonary, surgical and trauma ICU.

CRITICAL PATHS/PATHWAYS

Clinical management tools that organize, sequence, and time the major interventions of nursing staff, physicians and other departments for a particular case type, subset or condition.

CRITICALLY ILL PATIENT

A patient who is at high risk for an actual or potential life-threatening health problem and that requires intense and vigilant nursing care.

CROSSOVER CLAIM

When claim information is sent from a primary insurance carrier to a secondary insurance carrier, or vice versa.

C-SUITE

A widely used slang term used as a collective reference to the Chief Officers of the hospital such as the Chief Executive Officer, Chief Operating Officer, Chief Nursing Officer etc.

CT SCANNER

A computerized tomographic (CT) scanner is a diagnostic tool that utilizes a beam of X-rays and a computer to generate thin cross-sectional images of the head, neck, chest, abdomen and extremities that are then displayed on a computer or transferred to film.

CUBIC CENTIMETER (CC)

A metric unit of volume equal to one-thousandth of a liter (a milliliter). One cubic centime is equal to 1 mL.

CULTURE

A laboratory test (within microbiology) that detects infections in the body by placing samples in special nutrients that allow bacteria to grow. A culture can also detect a sensitivity to antibiotics.

CURRENT ASSETS

Unrestricted cash, or other assets held for conversion into cash within a relatively short period or other readily convertible assets, or currently useful goods or services. The five categories of current assets are cash, temporary investments, receivables, inventory, and prepaid expenses.

CURRENT LIABILITY

A hospital's debt or obligations that are due within one year. Current liabilities appear on the hospital's balance sheet and include short term debt, accounts payable, accrued liabilities and other debts.

CURRENT PROCEDURAL TERMINOLOGY (CPT)

This is a set of codes that is used to report medical procedures and services to physicians, health insurance companies and accreditation organizations. CPT is used in conjunction with ICD-9-CM or ICD-10-CM numerical diagnostic coding during the electronic medical billing process.

CURRENT RATIO

Ratio of current assets to current liabilities. Used as the basic index of liquidity and financial position.

CUSHION RATIO

A measure of the capital structure of the organization. It is calculated by taking the cash equivalents plus the board designated amounts for capital divided by the estimated future peak debt service. This ratio is important in evaluating the financial risk position of an organization.

CUSTODIAL CARE

Non-skilled service or non-medical care, such as help with bathing, dressing, eating, getting in and out of bed or chair, moving around, using the bathroom and the preparation of special diets. Providers of custodial care are not required to undergo medical training.

CUSTOMARY CHARGE

One of the factors that is used to determine a physician's payment for services rendered under Medicare.

CUSTOMARY, PREVAILING AND REASONABLE (CPR)

The method by which physicians are paid by Medicare. Physician services are paid the lowest of their billed charge, the physician's customary charge or the prevailing charge for that service within the community.

CUSTOM PROCEDURE TRAY (CPT)

Sterile trays that are customized to the surgeon's preference for a surgical procedure.

CYANOSIS

A bluish or gray discoloration of the skin caused by insufficient oxygen.

CYCLE COUNT

A scheduled, periodic count of all on-hand supplies.

CYTOGENETICS

Services provided that relate to the study of chromosomes.

CYTOLOGY

The medical and scientific study of cells. Cytology is a branch of pathology that examines tissue samples from the body and helps in the diagnosis of diseases.

CYSTOSCOPE

A flexible tube containing a fiber-optic cable with a light and a camera lens at the end to view the inside of the urethra and bladder cavity.

CYTOSOCOPY

A procedure that examines the inside of the urethra and bladder cavity with a cystoscope.

DAILY HOSPITAL SERVICES

Those inpatient services generally included by the hospital in a daily service charge - sometimes referred to as the "room and board" charge.

DAILY INPATIENT CENSUS

The number of inpatients present at the census time each day, plus any inpatients who were admitted and discharged or died after the census-taking time the previous day. Generally, the inpatient census is taken each midnight.

DATA BREACH

When sensitive, protected or confidential data has been stolen, potentially viewed or used by an individual unauthorized to do so. Within healthcare data breaches most often involve personal health information (PHI).

DATA CENTRE

The physical location where a healthcare organization's data are stored. Many are stored off-site in data warehouses or centres.

DATA CLUSTERING

The grouping of related data.

DATA COLLECTION

In a research project it is the gathering of information and the identification of the sampling method used.

DATA COMPARISON REPORTING SYSTEM (DCRS)

A national comparative database designed to help identify ways a hospital can improve its financial and operational performance. Departmental productivity can be compared with other hospitals.

DATA ENCRYPTION

The codifying of information into an unreadable state using algorithms or ciphers. This process plays a key role in the secure transmission of information, such as patient data.

DATA GOVERNANCE

Focuses on structured data such as the quality, security and ownership of the data and how the data is shared.

DATA MINING

The process of analyzing large amounts of data and looking for patterns that are statistically significant and therefore meaningful. They are used to make better decisions about the future.

DATA RETRIEVAL

The recovery of information from the source used i.e. database, manual or Excel files etc.

DATA WAREHOUSE

A repository of data that is organized in a format that is suitable for query processing as it is required.

DATE OF ACQUISITION

The effective purchase date of an asset. Usually, this is the date title is acquired and the asset is in possession.

DATE OF BIRTH (DOB)

The date a patient was born.

DATE OF SERVICE

The date(s) that health care services were provided to the beneficiary.

DAYS CASH ON HAND

A financial calculation of how many days a healthcare facility can continue to pay its daily cash obligations without receiving any new revenue.

DAYS IN ACCOUNTS RECEIVABLE

The average number of days it takes to collect payment for services rendered.

DAYS OF SUPPLY

A measure of the quantity of inventory-on-hand, in relation to number of days of projected usage.

DAYS SALES OUTSTANDING (DSO)

The average number of days it takes for a receivable to be paid.

DEAD ON ARRIVAL (DOA)

A designation given to products which are not functional when delivered. Also called Out-of-Box Failures.

DEBRIDEMENT

The process of removing dead tissue (which may be black, gray, yellow, tan or white) from wounds.

DEBRIEF

Unsuccessful bidders may be entitled to a debrief meeting with the procurement buyer and/or end user to discuss the results of the solicitation process.

DEDUCTIBLE

The monetary amount a patient must pay for covered healthcare before the insurance company pays the balance.

DEDUCTIONS FROM REVENUE

The difference between gross patient revenue (charges based on full established rates) and amounts received from patients and third-party payers for services performed. Deductions from revenue can include contractual adjustments, bad debts, and charity care.

DEFAULT

Failure to pay debt services when due.

DELIVERY TERMS

Conditions in a contract relating to freight charges, place of delivery, time of delivery or method of transportation.

DEMAND MANAGEMENT

The formal process of determining the hospitals anticipated demand requirements compared to the supply chains capabilities to ensure uninterrupted supply.

DEMOGRAPHIC TRENDS

The results of a study of measurable population data such as age, race, sex, economic status, level of education, income level, employment etc.

DEMURRAGE CHARGES

The payment required and made for the delay of a ship, railroad, car or truck beyond a specified time for loading and unloading.

DENIAL DAYS

The number of hospital inpatient days which have been determined to be medically not necessary.

DENIAL OF CLAIM

The refusal by a third-party payer to reimburse a provider for services or a refusal to authorize payment for services prospectively. Denials are generally issued on the basis that a hospital admission, diagnostic test, treatment or continued stay is inappropriate according to a set of guidelines.

DEPARTMENT

Any cost center of a hospital that employs personnel.

DEPARTMENT OF HEALTH & HUMAN SERVICES

The department within the federal government which oversees all things health and human services related. They administer and regulate all federal regulations and attempt to enhance the health of individuals through the provision of various social services.

DEPENDENT

An individual or individuals that rely on the policy holder for support. This may include the spouse and/or unmarried children (whether natural, adopted or step) of an insured.

DEPRECIABLE COST

That part of the capitalized cost of a fixed asset that is to be spread over its useful life.

DEPRECIATION

Lost usefulness or expired utility from a fixed asset that cannot or will not be restored by repairs or by replacement of parts.

DERMATOLOGY

The branch of medicine that studies, diagnoses and treats diseases of the skin, nails and hair.

DERMATOLOGY CLINIC

The out-patient services that relate to the diagnosis and treatment of skin disorders.

DIABETES CLINIC

Services that relate to the out-patient diagnosis and treatment of a patient with diabetes.

DIABETES TRAINING CLASS

Instruction provided to individuals for their treatment of diabetes.

DIAGNOSIS (DX)

The determination of the cause of a patient's illness or complaint through patient interviews, physical examination, laboratory tests and review of the patient's medical records.

DIAGNOSIS-RELATED GROUP (DRG)

A system of classification for inpatient hospital services based on principle diagnosis, secondary diagnosis, surgical procedures, age, sex and presence of complications. This classification system is used as a financing mechanism to reimburse hospital and selected other providers for services rendered. Hospitals receive a set dollar amount, determined in advance, based on the length of time patients with a given diagnosis are likely to stay in the hospital. Also called Prospective Payment System (PPS).

DIAGNOSTIC IMAGING EQUIPMENT

All of the devices that are used for the visualization and study of the human body.

DIAGNOSTIC IMAGING SERVICES

The use of imaging equipment to assist a doctor in diagnosis. Examples include an MRI, CT Scanner etc.

DIAGNOSTIC TESTS

Tests and procedures ordered by a physician to determine if the patient has a certain condition or disease based upon specific signs or symptoms demonstrated by the patient. These diagnostic tests include but are not limited to radiology, ultrasound, nuclear medicine, laboratory or pathology services.

DIALYSIS

The process of cleansing the blood by passing it through a mechanical filter. Dialysis is necessary when the kidneys are not able to filter the blood properly. Most patients begin dialysis when their kidneys have lost 85%-90% of their ability. A patient may be on dialysis for a short time, or may need it for the rest of their life (or until they receive a kidney transplant), depending on the reason for the kidney failure.

DIALYSIS MACHINE

A machine that functions as an artificial kidney. It filters a patient's blood and removes excess water and waste products. It is used when the kidneys are damaged or missing.

DIETARY SERVICES DEPARTMENT

The Department that oversees food and meal preparation for patients in the hospital. Registered dietitians contribute to the patient's treatment plan by recommending which hospital diet to prescribe. The meals are balanced and personalized with regard to patient preferences and intolerances/allergies. Registered dietitians also instruct hospitalized patients on diet and monitor the effectiveness of their nutrition care plan. Patients discharged from the hospital may receive follow-up diet consultation on an outpatient basis. Also called Food & Nutrition Services Department.

DIETETIC COUNSELLING

Counselling services provided around the proper planning and preparation of foods to adhere to a diet for both health and disease reasons.

DIFFERENTIAL DIAGNOSIS

The process of differentiating between two or more conditions that share similar signs or symptoms in order to determine a patient's condition.

DIGITAL PATHOLOGY:

The system engaged in the digitalization, storage, transmission and display of glass slide images.

DILATOR

An instrument used for enlarging an opening or cavity such as the cervix, the male urethra, or the rectum. Dilators also are used to widen a punctured opening for easier insertion of invasive applications such as catheters.

DIRECT ACCESS

The ability of a patient to see a physician or receive a medical service without a referral from a primary care physician.

DIRECT ADMISSION

An admission into the hospital usually scheduled in advance from a doctor's office, clinic, or the emergency department. These patients usually have a room/bed reserved.

DIRECT COST

The cost of any good or service that is attributable to product or service output.

DIRECT EXPENSE

The cost of any good or service that contributes to (and is readily attributable to) the hospital's product or service output.

DIRECT HOURS

Hands on patient care hours.

DIRECT SERVICE NURSES

The number of nurses providing hands –on patient care. This does not include agency nurses.

DIRECTED (SINGLE) SOURCE

The purchase of any commodities or services, regardless of amount, where it can be substantiated that only one vendor or contractor provides a good or service that is distinguishable from others in the market place and singularly meets all significant elements of the business requirement.

DISALLOWANCE

A denial by a health care payer for all or some portion of the claimed amount.

DISASTER DRILL

A periodic exercise that tests the hospitals or healthcare facility's readiness and capacity to respond to a public health emergency or local disaster.

DISASTER PLAN

A disaster is an unplanned event in which the needs of the affected community outweigh the available resources. This can be internal such as a fire, explosion or a shooting or external such as a tornado or hurricane, an airline crash, bombing etc. When these untoward events occur hospitals need special planning for both, mass accident admissions as well as damage area management. Every hospital has a disaster plan in place that is tested periodically.

DISCHARGE

A discharge from the hospital is when the patient leaves the hospital and either returns home or is transferred to another facility such as one for rehabilitation or to a skilled nursing facility. This term excludes births and transfers within the facility.

DISCHARGE DAYS

The total number of days between the admission and discharge dates for each patient (length of stay).

DISCHARGE HOUR

The time of day when a patient was discharged from a hospital or health care facility.

DISCHARGE PLANNING

Centralized, coordinated program developed by a hospital to ensure that each patient has a planned program for follow-up care after discharge from the hospital.

DISCHARGES

The total number of patients discharged from a hospital acute care bed in a given time period. Discharges are often reported by payor type.

DISCHARGE SUMMARY

The clinical report that is prepared at the end of a patient's hospital stay or series of out-patient treatments.

DISCOUNT

The amount that the list price is reduced by the seller to try and encourage purchase of the product or service.

DISCOUNT EARNED

A reduction in the purchase price of a good or service because of early payment.

DISEASE MANAGEMENT

Refers to the process of a physician managing a patient's disease (such as diabetes or COPD) on a long-term, continuing basis, rather than treating a single episode.

DISINTERMEDIATION

The removal of any intermediary in a supply chain; i.e. "to cut out the middleman" and deal directly with the source for the product, service or solution. For example, an agreement to purchase directly from a manufacturer instead of through a distributor.

DISPROPORTIONATE SHARE HOSPITAL (DSH)

A hospital that provides care to a large number of patients who cannot afford to pay or do not have insurance. Reimbursement is at a higher rate under the prospective payment system for inpatient services to cover the higher cost of caring for these patients. Inner city and rural hospitals typically fall into this category.

DISPROPORTIONATE SHARE HOSPITAL (DSH) ADJUSTMENT

An additional payment under Medicare or Medicaid to hospitals that serve a relatively large volume of low-income patients.

DISPROPORTIONATE SHARE HOSPITAL (DSH) PAYMENT

Specific federal compensation to hospitals that serve a significantly higher number of low-income Medicaid and/or Medicare patients.

DISTRIBUTION

An organization or layer of organizations that make a product or service available for use by a hospital or healthcare facility. Typically a distributor will purchase the item(s), provide sales and service and resell the product directly to the hospital or healthcare facility.

DISTRIBUTION CENTER

The warehouse facility which holds inventory from a manufacturer or distributor pending distribution to the hospital or a department/location within the hospital.

DISTRIBUTOR

An organization that usually does not manufacture its own products, but purchases and resells products.

DIURETIC

A substance that removes water from the body through urination and the loss of sale (sodium).

DOCTOR OF MEDICINE (MD)

Doctor of Medicine is one of two doctoral degrees that are granted by USA medical schools. The other is the Doctor of Osteopathy (DO).

DOCTOR OF OSTEOPATHY (DO)

Doctor of Osteopathy is one of two doctoral degrees that are granted by USA medical schools. The other is the Doctor of Medicine (MD).

DO NOT RESUSCITATE (DNR)

A written directive to not attempt manual or mechanical resuscitation if the patient stops breathing.

DOSE

The amount of a drug or other substance to be given to a patient at a particular time or frequency.

DOUBLE BLIND STUDY

A study in which neither the patient nor the researcher knows if the patient is receiving the treatment or a placebo.

DRAINAGE TUBE

A catheter that evacuates air or fluid from a cavity or wound.

DRUG

A chemical compound used to prevent, diagnose, or treat an individual's condition.

DRUG FORMULARY

A listing of prescription medications that are approved for use by a hospital and which will be dispensed through the pharmacy.

DRUG UTILIZATION REVIEW

A quantitative evaluation of prescription drug use, physician prescribing patterns or patient drug utilization to determine the appropriateness of drug therapy.

DURABLE MEDICAL EQUIPMENT (DME)

Devices which are very resistant to wear and may be used over an extended period of time. DME includes items such as walkers, wheelchairs, hospital beds, oxygen concentrators etc.

DURABLE POWER OF ATTORNEY FOR HEALTH CARE

A legal document that allows an individual to designate in advance another person to act on his/her behalf if he/she is unable to make a decision to accept, maintain, discontinue, or refuse any health care services.

E-COMMERCE

Business that is conducted online. This may include buying, selling, service and more.

EAR, NOSE AND THROAT (ENT)

A physician that specializes in the diagnosis and treatment of disorders of the head and neck, both medically and surgically; for the ears, nose and throat.

ECHOCARDIOGRAPHY

A diagnostic test of the heart that uses ultrasound waves to show the chambers, valves and structures of the heart. It is used to detect inflammation, infections and abnormal anatomy of the heart.

ECONOMIC INCENTIVES

Initiatives to reward and motivate healthcare providers who provide effective and efficient care using specific performance measures.

ECONOMIC ORDER QUANTITY (EOQ)

A fixed order entry model that determines the amount of an item to be purchased at one time. The goal is to minimize the combined costs of acquiring product and carrying inventory.

ECONOMIC VALUE ADDED (EVA)

A financial measure that subtracts the capital charge (the capital investment times the cost of capital) from the net financial benefits of the investment.

ECONOMIES OF SCALE

A decrease in unit costs because of the volume purchased.

EFFECTIVE DATE OF AWARD

The date the contract will start.

EFFECTIVENESS

The degree to which patient care is provided correctly according to the current state of clinical knowledge, to achieve the desired or projected outcome(s) for the patient.

ELDER ABUSE

Any intentional or negligent act by a caregiver or any other person that causes harm or a serious risk of harm to a vulnerable older adult (usually disabled or frail). Types of elder abuse may include physical, emotional or sexual abuse, neglect, exploitation or abandonment.

ELDER CARE

Care for aged individuals. It is also commonly referred to as geriatric care or senior care, and includes a wide range of care services, including help with ADLs.

ELECTIVE

A healthcare procedure that is not an emergency and that the patient and doctor plan in advance.

ELECTIVE ADMISSION

An admission that can be scheduled because the illness or injury is not life threatening. An example is hip or knee surgery.

ELECTIVE SURGERY

Surgery that is scheduled in advance because it does not involve a medical emergency.

ELECTROCARDIOGRAM (ECG OR EKG)

Measures the electrical activity of the heart. The heart generates an electrical signal which flows out from the heart through the body. Small electrical sensors, called electrodes, are put on the skin to sense the electricity that began in the heart. The electrical activity is then turned into a graph. This can give doctors an idea of whether the heart is beating normally.

ELECTRON BEAM COMPUTED TOMOGRAPHY

A high-tech computed tomography scan used to detect coronary artery disease by measuring coronary calcifications.

ELECTROENCEPHALOGRAM (EEG)

A noninvasive and painless study, in which electrodes are placed on the scalp to record the electrical currents of the brain.

ELECTRONIC CLAIM

When the claims data is submitted directly from one computer to another. This requires that claims data be entered into a computer system and followed by a telephone call to the insurance carrier's computer system using a modem.

ELECTRONIC DATA INTERCHANGE (EDI)

The mutual communication or exchange of business documents between two entities using a standardized format via computer

ELECTRONIC HEALTH RECORD (EHR)

Computerized patient health records, including medical, demographic and administrative information that can be shared across multiple healthcare facilities and physicians for overall continuity in care. It is an aggregate of a patient's health information and is more comprehensive than the information collected by a physician in his/her office through an electronic medical record (EMR).

ELECTRONIC MEDICAL RECORD (EMR)

An electronic medical record is a record of patient health maintained by the patient's physician as a record of that physician's care of the patient.

ELECTRONIC PROTECTED HEALTH INFORMATION (EPHI)

Any individually identifiable health information that is created, maintained or transmitted electronically.

ELECTRONIC REQUISITIONING

An electronic method of submitting supply requests to purchasing or a distribution center by the hospital department or functional area.

ELECTRONIC TENDERING

A computer based system that provides suppliers with access to information related to open competitive procurements.

EMERGENCY ADMISSION

An admission into the hospital because of an accident or a medical emergency through the Emergency Department.

EMERGENCY CARE

Any health care service that is provided in an emergency facility or setting after the onset of an illness or medical condition that without immediate medical attention could place the individual in physical and or mental health jeopardy.

EMERGENCY DEPARTMENT (ED)

The department responsible for evaluating the medical needs of emergency and non-emergency cases entering it and determining the appropriate treatment. The Emergency Department takes care of people of all ages. Service is provided 24 hours a day.

EMERGENCY DEPARTMENT (ED) CARE

Emergency services received in an emergency room. May also be called Emergency Room care.

EMERGENCY DEPARTMENT (ED) LENGTH OF STAY

The measurement from ED arrival time to ED departure time.

EMERGENCY DEPARTMENT (ED) VISITS

The total number of patient visits to the emergency department.

EMERGENCY DEPARTMENT (ED) WAIT TIME

The amount of time a patient waits until they are seen by an a licensed provider (doctor, physician assistant or nurse practitioner).

EMERGENCY HELICOPTER SERVICE

Air transportation services provided for individuals that require urgent medical care.

EMERGENCY MEDICAL SERVICES (EMS) VISITS:

Visits made during the year to the Emergency Medical Service (EMS) or Emergency Department (ED). These visits are classified in the following three categories:

- **NON-URGENT**

  a patient with a non-emergent injury, illness, or condition; sometimes chronic; that can be treated in a non-emergency setting and not necessarily on the same day they are seen in the EMS-ED department (e.g., laboratory tests, minor cold, chest x-ray).

- **URGENT**

  a patient with an acute injury or illness where loss of life or limb is not an immediate threat to their well-being, or a patient who needs a timely evaluation (possible fracture or a laceration).

- **CRITICAL**

  a patient presents an acute injury or illness that could result in permanent damage, injury or death (head injury, vehicular accident, a shooting).

EMERGENCY MEDICAL TRANSPORTATION

Ambulance or fire department services provided for an emergency medical condition.

EMERGENCY MEDICINE

A physician who specializes in the area of emergency medicine. The emergency physician's role is to assess; treat, admit, or discharge any patient that seeks medical attention. They take a full patient history, perform a physical exam, and order and obtain the tests necessary to ascertain the cause of the patient's complaint. Upon making a diagnosis, the physician must either treat the patient or refer him/her for the appropriate follow up care. A trained emergency physician is able to handle traumas and acute and non-acute problems.

EMS-ED VISITS RESULTING IN ADMISSIONS

Emergency Medical Services-ED visits that result in hospital admissions.

EMPLOYEE

An individual that is on the payroll of the hospital and whose employment is subject to the hospitals will and control.

EMPLOYEE BENEFIT

Any tangible benefit such as insurance coverage, paid vacation, holidays, sick days or other costs which are not paid for by the employee.

EMPLOYEE BENEFIT EXPENSE

Fringe benefits and other non-payroll expenditures that benefit the employee.

EMPLOYEES, FULL-TIME

Number of individuals on the hospital payroll at the end of the reporting period who work at least 35 hours per week.

EMPLOYEES, PART-TIME

Number of individuals on the hospital payroll at the end of the reporting period who work less than 35 hours per week.

EMPLOYEES, TOTAL

Number of individuals on the hospital payroll at the end of the reporting period.

EMPLOYER-BASED HEALTH CARE

Refers to health plans that are offered at the workplace for employees.

EMPLOYER IDENTIFICATION NUMBER (EIN)

The number assigned to the provider by the federal government for tax reporting purposes. Also known as the Federal Tax Number or Tax Identification Number (TIN).

ENCOUNTER

A face-to-face meeting between an individual and a health care provider where services are provided or rendered.

ENCOUNTER DATA

The description of the diagnosis made and services provided when a patient visits a health care provider.

ENDOCRINOLOGY

The study of hormones and diseases and conditions associated with hormonal imbalance.

ENDOSCOPE

An instrument used to look inside an organ or body cavity. It is comprised of composed of a fiber-optic cable for visualization or recording (camera), a light source and a lumen to take samples of the area being viewed.

ENDOSCOPY

The use of instrumentation for direct visual inspection of a hollow organ or cavity with an endoscope.

ENDOTRACHEAL

Refers to within the trachea. An endotracheal tube is an airway catheter which is inserted into the trachea when a patient requires ventilatory support.

ENDOTRACHEAL TUBE (ETT OR ET TUBE)

A tube placed through the mouth or nose into the trachea (airway). This tube provides a secure pathway through which oxygen can be circulated to the lungs.

END STAGE DISEASE

A disease that is terminal or not reversible.

ENDOWMENT FUND

Funds intended to be invested in perpetuity, providing income for the continued support of a not-for-profit organization (hospital). The income can be used for a specific purpose or at the institutions discretion as specified by the donor.

ENGINEERING AND MAINTENANCE

Provides for maintenance of the hospital's physical plant, including heating, ventilating and air conditioning systems, utilities, telecommunications and clinical engineering equipment.

ENROLLEE

A person who is covered by health insurance.

ENTERAL

Within the gastrointestinal tract. Patient feeding is often accomplished through a naso-gastric tube.

ENTERPRISE RESOURCE PLANNING (ERP) SYSTEMS

The name given for a software systems used by hospitals or health systems to manage and plan resources, including human resources, payroll, customer accounts and their supply chain.

ENVIRONMENTAL SERVICES

The hospital department that provides for maintenance of a safe and sanitary hospital by controlling solid and liquid wastes, radiation exposure and pathogenic organisms. The department also handles the daily cleaning routine, scheduled project work such as window washing and floor waxing, and cleaning of patient rooms during and after a patient's stay in the hospital. Also called Housekeeping Department.

EPIDURAL CATHETER

A catheter inserted in the lower back that is often used for the injection of a local analgesic in order to block the spinal nerves during labor or surgery.

E-PRESCRIPTION

Prescriptions that are sent electronically from providers to pharmacies for patients to pick up without the need for telephone calls or paper prescriptions.

ETHICS COMMITTEE

Hospital Committee concerned with biomedical ethics issues. Its purpose may be to direct educational programs or provide forums for discussion of ethics issues among hospital medical professionals and others, to serve in an advisory capacity and/or as a resource to healthcare professionals involved in biomedical ethical implications.

ETIOLOGY

The study of all of the causes that may be involved in the development of a disease.

EVALUATION COMMITTEE

A committee that advises and assists the purchasing activity. This committee may be called the value analysis committee, technology committee, new product committee etc.

EVALUATION COMMITTEE LEAD

The individual in charge of the evaluation committee and that coordinates the team's progress.

EVALUATION CRITERIA

A benchmark, standards or yardstick against which bid suppliers and proposals can be evaluated.

EVALUATION MATRIX

An objective tool that allows the evaluation committee to rate each potential supplier based upon multiple predefined criteria in an objective and fair manner.

EVIDENCE-BASED MEDICINE

The wise and careful use of the best available scientific research and practices with proven effectiveness in daily medical decision making, including individual clinical practice decisions, by well-trained, experienced clinicians. This approach must balance the best external evidence with the desires of the patient and the clinical expertise of health care providers.

EXCESS CAPACITY

The difference between the number of hospital beds being used for patient care and the number of beds available.

EXCESS MARGIN %

Total operating revenue plus non-operating revenue minus total operating expenses divided by total operating revenue plus non-operating expenses. This measure is often preferred over the operating margin because it includes all sources of income and expenses.

EXCESS OR STAFFING COSTS

Measures the staffing costs associated with underused and overused OR time.

EXCLUDED SERVICES

Health care services that an individual's health insurance or plan doesn't pay for or cover under the plan.

EXCLUSION CRITERIA

Any factors that prevent an individual from participating in a clinical trial.

EXCLUSIONS

To omit from consideration.

EXCHANGE CART

A supply cart in which identical items are kept at identical supply levels. During the restocking process the carts are physically exchanged for each other. This leaves a fully stocked cart while the previous cart is being refilled.

EXEMPTIONS

Free from duty or obligation required by others.

EXISTING PURCHASE ORDER

An order that has been set up in the hospital system against a requisition.

EXPECTED LIFE

The expected length of life in years of service of an asset used by the hospital or healthcare facility.

EXPENSES TOTAL

All of the expenses for the reporting period including payroll, non-payroll, bad debt and all other expenses.

EXPERIMENTAL TREATMENT

A type of treatment that is still under medical study as a clinical trial and is not accepted by the general medical community and professional medical organizations and is not approved by the FDA.

EXPLANATION OF BENEFITS (EOB) OR EXPLANATION OF MEDICAL BENEFITS (EOMB)

The written notice received by a patient from their insurance company after receiving medical services from a doctor or hospital. It outlines what was billed, the payment amount that was approved by insurance, the amount paid, and the amount to pay for services rendered.

EXTENDED-CARE FACILITY

A facility or a distinct part of a facility that provides skilled nursing care and rehabilitation services to residents that do not require hospital care.

EXTENDED RELEASE MEDICINES

Medications that are slowly released into the body to reduce how fast the body absorbs the medicine. Also called modified-release, prolonged release, controlled-release, controlled delivery, slow release and sustained-release medicines.

EXTRACORPOREAL MEMBRANE OXYGENATOR (ECMO)

The name means "oxygenation outside the body." It's an external mechanical device that oxygenates a patient's blood outside the body and then returns the blood to the patient's circulatory system.

EXTREMELY LOW BIRTH WEIGHT

Babies with a birth weight of less than 1,000 g or 2 lbs. 3 oz.

FACP

The designation given for members that a Fellow of the American College of Chest Physicians.

FACS

The designation given for members that are a Fellow of the American College of Surgeons.

FACE SHEET

A form included in the inpatient medical record that contains personal and demographic information. It is developed by the Admitting department.

FACILITIES MANAGEMENT

The department responsible for keeping all the utilities; including heating, cooling, ventilation, plumbing and electrical working properly 24 hours a day, 7 days a week, 365 days a year. They are also responsible for responding to everyday work orders and whatever building projects may be necessary throughout the year.

FALSE CLAIMS ACT

A law that establishes civil liability for offenses related to certain acts, such as knowingly presenting a false or fraudulent claim to the federal government for payment.

FALSE NEGATIVE

A test result that indicates the condition of interest is not present when in fact it is present. An example is when a test comes back negative for pregnancy but the patient is pregnant.

FALSE POSITIVE

A test result that indicates the condition of interest is present when in fact it is not present. An example is when a test comes back positive for pregnancy but the patient is not pregnant.

FAMILY PRACTICE/FAMILY MEDICINE (FP)

The medical specialty that provides continuous and comprehensive primary care for all members of the family, regardless of age or sex.

FDA CLASS I MEDICAL DEVICES

Devices that present minimal potential harm to the patient, and are not life-supporting or life-sustaining (e.g., tongue depressors, bedpans, or examination gloves). These medical devices are simpler in design than Class II and III devices and are only subject to general federal controls that are deemed sufficient to provide reasonable assurance of the safety and effectiveness of the device.

FDA CLASS II MEDICAL DEVICES

Devices that are held to a higher level of assurance that they will perform as indicated and will not cause injury or harm to the patient (e.g., x-ray machines, surgical needles, or suture materials). Class II devices are subject to special controls, in addition to the general controls of Class I devices, which may include labeling requirements, mandatory performance standards, and post-market surveillance.

FDA Class III Medical Devices

Devices for which insufficient information exists to assure safety and effectiveness solely through the general or special controls applied to Class I or Class II devices (e.g., replacement heart valves, implanted cerebral stimulators, or implantable pacemaker pulse generators). Class III devices require pre-market approval.

Federal Fiscal Year (FFY)

The federal government's accounting year, which begins October 1 and ends September 30.

Federal Poverty Level (FPL)

The reference point established by the federal government that determines the number of people with income below the poverty level and income level for eligibility for subsidies on the Health Insurance Marketplace, and/or government-sponsored programs.

Federal Tax Number

The number assigned to the provider by the federal government for tax reporting purposes. Also known as the Tax Identification Number (TIN) or Employer Identification Number (EIN).

Federally Qualified Health Centers

Community health clinics and public housing centers that provide health care services regardless of the individual's ability to pay. These are funded by the federal government.

Fee Schedule

A list of the fees used to reimburse a physician and/or other provider on a fee-for-services basis which the physician agrees to accept as payment in full. While physicians typically charge fees per procedure, Medicare and other payors have a payment fee schedule per procedure that is typically less than that charged. Also known as a fee allowance, fee maximum or capped fee.

Fee-For-Service (FFS)

A system of health insurance payment in which a physician or other health care provider is paid a fee for each particular service rendered.

Fellow

A physician who has completed training as an intern and resident and has chosen to continue training toward a specialty.

FELLOWSHIP TRAINING

Postgraduate training for doctors in specialized fields. The training can include clinical (patient care) and research (laboratory) work. Additional training in a specialty which occurs at the conclusion of residency training.

FIDUCIARY

A fiduciary relationship exists where an individual or organization has an explicit or implicit obligation to act in behalf of another person's or organization's interests in matters which affect the other person or organization. A physician has such a relation with his/her patient, and a hospital trustee has one with a hospital.

FILL RATE

The percentage of line items on a purchase order that are successfully received from a supplier as compared to the total number of purchase order line items that were ordered.

FINANCIAL ANALYSIS

The interpretation of financial data in order to make a hospital more financially stable.

FINANCIAL ASSISTANCE

Assistance provided to patients who have financial hardship and therefore difficulty in paying their medical bill.

FINANCIAL CLASS

The classification assigned to a patient account by a health care provider, reflecting an expected method of payment (e.g., self-pay, Blue Cross, Medicaid, Commercial insurance, etc.).

FINANCIAL STATEMENT

Detailed report of the financial conditions of an entity including profits, losses, assets and liabilities. A balance sheet, income statement, funds statement, or any other statement of financial data derived from accounting documentation.

FIRST CASE START-TIME ACCURACY

This Operating Room key performance indicator measures the percentage of first cases of the day that start on time. It is typically defined as the patient being in the OR at the scheduled start time. Most facilities allow for a 15-minute grace period.

FIRST DOLLAR COVERAGE

Health care coverage that has no deductible provisions; thus the coverage starts with the first dollar of expense.

FIRST RESPONDER

The first medically trained person that arrives at the scene of an emergency to render care. This could be a police officer, firefighter or EMT.

FIRST YEAR RESIDENT

A physician (intern or resident) who has completed medical school, but is still undergoing the required training to be licensed to practice medicine independently. Also called an Intern.

FISCAL INTERMEDIARY (FI)

An organization that acts as an intermediary between the hospital and a third-party payer. It receives billings from the hospital and makes payments on behalf of the payer for covered services. It is, in turn, reimbursed by the third-party payer.

FISCAL YEAR (FY)

The hospital's accounting year.

FISCAL YEAR END

The last day of the hospital's accounting period.

FIXED ASSET

A tangible asset held for the services it yields in the production of goods and services. Examples of hospital fixed assets are land, buildings, medical equipment, fixtures, furniture etc.

FLUID MANAGEMENT

The promotion of fluid balance and the prevention of complications from undesirable fluid levels.

FLUOROSCOPY

An X-ray procedure that makes it possible to see internal organs in motion.

F.O.B. (FREE ON BOARD)

Contractual terms between a buyer and a seller that define where title transfer takes place.

F.O.B. DESTINATION

A shipping term that indicates the seller must pay the freight cost to the destination. Title for the goods delivered does not pass until the merchandise reaches its destination. This means the seller assumes all risks for loss, or damage while the goods are in transit, except for the liability of the freight.

F.O.B. ORIGIN

A form of pricing in which the seller quotes prices from the point of shipment. Free-on-board (F.O.B.) means it is the buyer's responsibility to select the mode of transport.

FOLEY CATHETER

A tube that is inserted into the bladder to drain urine.

FOOT & ANKLE SURGERY

This is a sub-specialty of orthopedics and podiatry that deals with the treatment, diagnosis and prevention of disorders of the foot and ankle both surgical and non-surgical. An orthopedic foot and ankle surgeon typically has four years of college, four years of allopathic or osteopathic school, one year of surgical internship, 4-5 years of orthopedic training and an optional 1 year fellowship in foot and ankle surgery. Training for a podiatric foot and ankle surgeon consists of four years of college, four years of podiatric medical school and 3–4 years of a surgical residency.

FORECASTABLE DEMAND

A method of forecasting that uses historical usage to forecast future demand.

FORENSIC MEDICINE

The branch of medicine that uses medical knowledge to establish facts in civil and criminal cases.

FORMAL COMPETITION

Process of soliciting written, sealed bids from several suppliers. Formal competition generally requires that the solicitation be publicly advertised, through a medium such as the internet or newspaper, and bid responses are due at a specific time, and are held sealed until the due date and time, at which time they are opened, reviewed and evaluated through a process managed by the buyer, with participation from the customer.

FORMAL SEALED BID

A bid that has been submitted in a sealed manner, either manually or electronically, to prevent its contents being revealed or known before the deadline for submission of all bids.

FORMULARY

The list of prescription medications that may be dispensed by the hospital. The formulary is selected based on the effectiveness of the drug, as well as its cost. The physician is requested or required to use only formulary drugs unless there is a valid medical reason to use a non-formulary drug.

FOR-PROFIT HOSPITAL (FP HOSPITAL)

A hospital that is owned and operated by a corporation or a group of investors. The initial source of funding is typically through the sale of stock; profits are paid to stockholders in dividends. These hospitals are also referred to as a proprietary or investor-owned hospitals. For profit hospitals pay income taxes.

FREE-STANDING ED (FSED)

A healthcare facility that is structurally separate and distinct from a hospital that provides emergency care. There are two distinct types of FSEDs

- A hospital outpatient department (HOPD), which is also referred to as an off-site hospital-based or satellite emergency department.

- Independent freestanding emergency centers (IFECs).

HOPDs are owned and operated by medical centers or hospital systems while IFECs are owned, in whole or in part, by independent groups or by individuals. As of this writing, CMS does not recognize IFECs as EDs which means that they don't allow for Medicare or Medicaid payment for the technical component of services provided by these facilities.

The American College of Emergency Physicians (ACEP) believes that any FSED facility whether it is an HOPD or an IFEC, should:

- Be open to the public 24 hours a day, seven days a week, 365 days per year.

- Be staffed by qualified emergency physicians and by a registered nurse (RN) at all times. As a minimum requirement the RN must have a current certification in advanced cardiac life support and pediatric advanced life support.

- Have adequate medical and nursing personnel that are qualified in emergency care to meet the emergency needs and procedures anticipated by the facility.

- Have an ability to provide effective and efficient transfer to a higher level of care if needed (i.e., cath labs, surgery, ICU).

FREESTANDING HOSPITAL
A hospital that is not formally tied to any other hospital or healthcare organization.

FRAUD AND ABUSE
Federal laws which prohibit the filing of false claims, paying or receiving kickbacks or bribes for referrals and self-referrals under the Medicare and Medicaid programs. Violations can result in criminal and civil penalties.

FTE LEAKAGE
The number of hours an individual has not worked but should have based upon their commitment to work full-time. This leakage often occurs when a manager allows paid time off without a replacement.

FULL-TIME EQUIVALENT (FTE)
A method for standardizing the number of full and part-time employees working in a hospital. A full-time employee working a 40-hour week, 52 weeks a year (2,080 hours/year) is equal to one full-time equivalent (FTE) and an employee who works for 20 hours per week is equal to 0.5 FTEs.

FULLY APPROVED
A term used within hospital procurement to indicate everyone in the approval process has approved the transaction.

FUND
A self-contained accounting entity set up to account for a specific activity or project.

GAIN SHARING
The legal sharing of profits based upon the utilization of lower cost effective treatments.

GENERAL ICU
The most common ICU found in hospitals and it usually encompasses patients that require medical and surgical intensive care.

GENERALLY ACCEPTED ACCOUNTING PRINCIPLES (GAAP)
A widely accepted set of rules, conventions, standards, and procedures for reporting financial information that was established by the Financial Accounting Standards Board.

GENERAL ANESTHESIA

Anesthesia where the patient is put to sleep usually with an intravenous (IV) drug and then maintained with a gas, requiring the patient to breathe through a mask or tube. Major operations usually are performed this way.

GENERAL LEDGER

A detailed record of each financial transaction of the hospital.

GENERAL SURGERY

Covers a wide range of types of surgery and procedures on patients incurring minimal invasive techniques.

GENERIC DRUG

A drug which is the pharmaceutical equivalent to one or more brand name drugs. Generic drugs have been approved by the Food and Drug Administration as meeting the same standards of safety, purity, strength, dosage, form and effectiveness as the brand name drug.

GENERIC SUBSTITUTION

Dispensing a generic drug in place of a brand name medication. Generic drugs are copies of brand-name drugs and are the same in dosage form, safety, strength, route of administration, quality, performance characteristics and intended use.

GENETIC DISORDERS

Diseases that can be passed from parents to their children. Some examples include: cystic fibrosis, sickle cell disease, Tay-Sachs disease, hemophilia and Duchenne muscular dystrophy

GENETICS

The hospital department that provides genetic services and testing for both children and adults. This includes risk assessment, evaluation, testing, and management as well as supportive counseling.

GERIATRIC

The treatment of the aged.

GERIATRIC CARE

Care for aged individuals. It is also commonly referred to as elder care or senior care, and includes a wide range of care services, including help with ADLs.

GERIATRIC MEDICINE

The medical specialty that focuses on the aging process and the diagnostic, therapeutic, preventive, and rehabilitative aspects of illness in the elderly. They typically provide care for geriatric patients in the patient's home, their office, in skilled nursing facilities and in the hospital. Examples of common geriatric conditions include incontinence, falls, Parkinson's disease and Alzheimer's disease.

GERONTOLOGY

The scientific study of, and learning about, the process of aging. It includes the social, cognitive, biological and psychological aspects.

GESTATION

The period of time between the last menstrual period and birth. Normal gestation is 40 weeks.

GIFT SHOP

The area of the hospital that carries a variety of gift items and seasonal merchandise. The gift shop is staffed by volunteers.

GOLDEN HOUR

It refers to a time period lasting for one hour, or less, following a medical emergency or traumatic injury, in which if patients get to a level 1 trauma center there is the highest likelihood that prompt medical treatment will prevent death. The "Golden Hour" was first described by R Adams Cowley, MD, at the University of Maryland Medical Center in Baltimore. It is based upon his personal experiences and observations in post-World War II Europe, and then in Baltimore in the 1960s.

GOVERNING BODY-BOARD

The legal entity ultimately responsible for hospital policy, organization, management, and quality of care. Also called the governing board, board of trustees, commissioners or directors. In Not-For-Profit Hospitals they are called a governing body and they are accountable to the owner(s) of the hospital, which is the community.

GRADUATE MEDICAL EDUCATION (GME)

Medical education after receipt of the doctor of medicine or equivalent degree, including the education received as an intern, resident or fellow, and continuing medical education.

GRAND ROUNDS

A formal meeting or lecture in which physicians discuss the clinical case of one or more patients to an audience consisting of doctors, residents and medical students. It is an important teaching tool within medical education and inpatient care. The intent of these sessions is to help doctors and other healthcare professionals keep up to date in important evolving areas of clinical acumen which may be outside of their core practice.

GREEN PROCUREMENT

The process of ensuring that the hospital or health system purchases environmentally preferable goods and services whenever possible. Performance considerations typically include reduced waste and support of reuse and recycling, improved energy and water efficiency, reduced hazardous waste etc.

GRIEVANCE

A complaint that you communicate in writing or verbally, to your health insurer or plan.

GROSS INPATIENT REVENUE

Gross revenue for daily hospital services and inpatient ancillary services before deductions from revenue are applied.

GROSS OUTPATIENT REVENUE

Gross revenue for outpatient ancillary services before deductions from revenue is applied.

GROSS PATIENT SERVICES REVENUE

The total charges at the hospital's full established rates for the provision of patient care services before deductions from revenue are applied.

GROSS REVENUE MEDICAID

Gross patient revenue from Medicaid.

GROSS REVENUE MEDICARE

Gross patient revenue from Medicare.

GROUP HEALTH INSURANCE

Insurance coverage offered through an employer or other entity that covers all individuals in the group.

GROUP HOME

These are private residential homes located within a community that are designed to provide housing, meals, housekeeping, personal care services to support children or adults with chronic disabilities. These homes usually have six or fewer occupants and are staffed 24 hours a day by trained caregivers. At least one caregiver is onsite at all times. In many states, group homes are licensed or certified and must meet criteria for facility safety, the types of services provided, and the number and type of residents they can provide care for.

GROUP PRACTICE

An association of three of more physicians and allied health professionals that provide health care services.

GROUP PURCHASING ORGANIZATION (GPO)

An entity that helps hospitals and other health care facilities realize savings and efficiencies by aggregating purchasing volume and using that leverage to negotiate discounted pricing with manufacturers, distributors and wholesalers.

GUARANTOR

The person responsible for paying the patient's bill. Typically, the guarantor is the patient's parent or guardian.

GYNECOLOGIC SURGERY

Gynecologic surgery includes Caesarean sections, hysterectomies, tubal ligation and other procedures involving the reproductive system. Caesarean sections (often referred to as "C-sections") occur when a woman is unable to deliver a baby vaginally. Many gynecologic surgeries can be performed laparoscopically, a minimally invasive procedure that results in faster recovery.

GYNECOLOGICAL SERVICES

Services provided for the treatment of diseases of the genital tract of women.

HAND SURGERY

The field of medicine that embodies the investigation, preservation and/or restoration of all structures of the upper extremity that support the form and function of the hand and wrist by medical, surgical or rehabilitative methods

HARD DATA

Information about a patient that is obtained by direct observation and measurement (laboratory and other diagnostic tests) instead of by interviewing the patient or other care-givers.

HCFA-1500 FORM

A health insurance claim form from the health care financing administration that is most commonly used when billing a) physician charges, b) independent laboratory charges, c) government programs, d) independent ambulance charges, e) durable medical equipment, f) CRNA/AA charges, and g) independent dialysis charges.

HEALTH & HUMAN SERVICES (HHS)

The department that administers all federal programs dealing with health and welfare in the U.S. The agency was started in 1979.

HEALTHCARE ASSOCIATED INFECTION (HAI)

An infection that a patient acquires while receiving treatment for another condition within a healthcare facility.

HEALTHCARE COST AND UTILIZATION PROJECT QUALITY INDICATORS (HCUP QIs)

Thirty three clinical performance measures of hospitals' self-assessment of their inpatient care along with state and community assessments of access to primary care. The 33 measures cover potentially avoidable adverse hospital outcomes, potentially inappropriate utilization of hospital resources and potentially avoidable hospital admissions.

HEALTHCARE GROWTH RATE

Is the percentage increase in the cost to treat patients from one year to the next. The projection is used by insurance companies to calculate health plan premiums for the coming year. The growth rate is influenced primarily by changes in the price of medical products and services, known as unit cost inflation and changes in the number of services used, or per capita utilization increases

HEALTHCARE PROVIDER

Someone who provides medical services, such as doctors, hospitals or laboratories.

HEALTH CARE SYSTEM

A corporate body that owns, leases and/or manages multiple entities including hospitals, long term care facilities, other institutional providers and programs, physician practices and/or insurance functions.

HEALTH ECONOMICS & OUTCOMES RESEARCH (HEOR)

Research that demonstrates clinical and economic evidence to providers, healthcare decision-makers and payers through clinical efficacy, real-world data, patient quality of life reports, opportunity cost of various treatment mixes, budget impact, and cost-effectiveness models.

HEALTH EDUCATION DEPARTMENT

The department that increases awareness of the importance of a healthy lifestyle and equips patients for optimal control over their health.

HEALTH FACILITY TRANSPORTATION

The service that offers patient transportation services to Physical Therapy, Occupational Therapy, Endoscopy etc.

HEALTH INFORMATION TECHNOLOGY (HEALTH IT; HIT)

The electronic management and exchange of comprehensive medical information between healthcare providers and patients.

HEALTH INSURANCE EXCHANGE-HEALTH INSURANCE MARKETPLACE

An online portal where consumers can shop for health insurance. Also known as a health insurance marketplace. All qualified plans must meet standards set by the Affordable Care Act (ACA).

HEALTH INSURANCE PORTABILITY AND ACCOUNTABILITY ACT (HIPPA)

A US law designed to provide privacy standards to protect patients' medical records and other health information provided to health plans, doctors, hospitals and other health care providers.

HEALTH LEVEL 7 (HL-7)

HL-7 is one of several standards setting organizations whose mission is to provide inter-operability standards for EHR systems.

HEALTH MAINTENANCE ORGANIZATION (HMO)

These are "pre-paid" or "capitated" insurance plans in which individuals or their employers pay a fixed monthly fee for services instead of a separate charge for each visit or service. The services are provided by physicians who are employed by, or under contract with, the HMO.

HEALTH OUTCOMES

The effect on health status from either the performance or non-performance of one or more processes or activities carried out by healthcare providers. Health outcomes typically include morbidity and mortality; physical, social, and mental functioning; nutritional status; etc.

HEALTH PERSONNEL

A generic term that includes all of the personnel that provide health care services.

HEALTH PLAN

An organization that offers reimbursement for its members' health-care services. It may be a health maintenance organization (HMO), a preferred provider organization (PPO), a commercial insurance carrier, or a company that self-insures.

HEART SURGERY

Any surgical procedure involving the heart.

HELIPORT

The physical location for helicopters to land.

HEMATOCRIT

The percentage of blood volume consisting of red blood cells. Low levels may indicate anemia as a result of bleeding, iron deficiency or the breakage of red blood cells while high levels may indicate chronic lung disease or other conditions.

HEMATOLOGY

The science or study of blood, blood-forming organs and blood diseases.

HEMOGLOBIN

The component of red blood cells that carries oxygen.

HEMOSTASIS

The body's natural physiologic response to prevent and stop bleeding. It is the first stage of wound healing. When hemostasis fails it leads to hemorrhage or blood clots (thrombosis)

HEPATITIS B VIRUS

A viral infection that attacks the liver and can cause both acute and chronic disease. The virus is transmitted through contact with the blood or other body fluids of an infected person.

HEPATOLOGY

The branch of medicine that studies the prevention, diagnosis and management of the liver, gall bladder, biliary tree and pancreas.

HIPAA AUDIT

A set of regulations, standards and implementation specifications by the Health Insurance Portability and Accountability Act.

HIPAA VIOLATIONS

The civil and criminal penalties that a company incurs if they fail to comply with Health Insurance Portability and Accountability Act (HIPAA) rules.

HISTOLOGY

The branch of science that deals with structure, composition, and function of cells and tissues.

HOLD HARMLESS

A clause frequently found in managed care contracts, whereby the HMO and the physician agree that neither will be held liable for malpractice or corporate malfeasance if either of the parties is found to be liable.

HOME CARE

Services provided by health professionals in an individual's place of residence on a per-visit or hourly basis to patients or clinics who have or are at risk of an injury, illness, or disabling conditions or who are terminally ill and require short-term or long-term interventions by health care professionals.

HOME HEALTH AGENCY (HHA)

An agency that provides home health care for individuals by matching a home health care professional with a patient in need of home health care.

HOME HEALTHCARE

Healthcare services that are provided in a patient's home. These often include nursing services, physical therapy services, occupational health services, speech and language therapy services, medical social services and home health visits.

HOME I.V. THERAPY SERVICES

Intravenous treatment provided to a patient at home.

HOME MONITORING

The use of technology to remotely monitor a patient's information from their home to enhance the patient's comfort, reduce costs and/or prevent hospitalization.

HOME NURSING CARE

Nursing care provided in the patient's home.

HOSPICE

A type of care for the terminally ill and their families in which treatment is geared to enable the patient to live as fully as possible, to relieve or control pain, to involve the family within the facility of care, and to provide the caring process in the home whenever possible.

HOSPICE CARE

A type of care that focuses on reducing the severity of a chronically ill, terminally ill, or seriously ill patient's pain and symptoms, and attending to their emotional needs. It is provided by a team of health care professionals and volunteers that provide medical, psychological, and spiritual support, often in a patient's home. The goal of the care is to help people who are dying have peace, comfort, and dignity while controlling their pain and other symptoms so they can remain as alert and comfortable as possible. Hospice programs also provide support services to a patient's family.

HOSPITAL

A health care institution with an organized medical and professional staff and with inpatient beds available around the clock. Its primary function is to provide inpatient medical, nursing and other health-related services to patients for both surgical and nonsurgical conditions. It also typically provides some outpatient services, particularly emergency care.

HOSPITAL CHARGE AUDIT

A post-payment service that can review medical claims before or after provider reimbursement.

HOSPITALIZATION

Care in a hospital that requires admission as an inpatient and requires an overnight stay.

HOSPITAL AFFILIATION

A contractual agreement between a health plan and one or more hospitals, such as an agreement for a hospital to provide the inpatient benefits offered by a health plan. May also refer to arrangements between hospitals and other health care financing or provider organizations.

HOSPITAL ALLIANCE

Agreements between hospitals to voluntarily join together on some services to reduce costs and achieve economies of scale.

HOSPITAL BASED PHYSICIAN

A physician who spends all or the majority of his/her time providing patient care services within a hospital instead of in an office setting.

HOSPITAL INDEMNITY POLICY

A policy that pays a fixed dollar amount for each day an individual is hospitalized, regardless of the actual costs.

HOSPITAL MANAGEMENT INFORMATION SYSTEM (HMIS)

Consists of computer software and hardware that a hospital or healthcare system uses to record data, process patient information and report operating information. It incorporates document management software, medical software and voice recognition applications.

HOSPITAL OUT-PATIENT CARE

Care in a hospital that usually doesn't require an overnight stay.

HOSPITAL UNIT

The hospital portion of a facility. It excludes physician offices, skilled nursing facilities etc. that may be attached to the facility.

HOUSEKEEPING DEPARTMENT

The hospital department that provides for maintenance of a safe and sanitary hospital by controlling solid and liquid wastes and pathogenic organisms. The department also handles the daily cleaning routine, scheduled project work such as window washing and floor waxing, and cleaning of patient rooms during and after a patient's stay in the hospital. Also called Environmental Services Department.

HOUSE STAFF

The aggregate body of physicians who have completed medical school and who participate in an accredited program of post-graduate medical education sponsored by a hospital (also called residents).

HUMAN IMMUNODEFICIENCY VIRUS

A virus that attacks the immune system.

HUMAN RESOURCES DEPARTMENT

The department that is responsible for the recruitment of new employees and retention of current employees. The responsibilities include employee relations, benefits administration, policy implementation, staffing and knowledge of all laws & regulations pertaining to human resources. Human Resources also act as a liaison between administration and staff assisting in the development of appropriate programs/plans in the resolution of the everyday business and workforce challenges.

HYBRID OPERATING ROOM

An operating room that has permanently installed equipment to enable diagnostic imaging before, during, and after a surgical procedure.

HYPERBARIC OXYGEN THERAPY

The use of a hyperbaric oxygen chamber to treat decompression sickness, carbon dioxide poisoning, gas gangrene, smoke inhalation, skin grafts or major burn injuries.

HYPERBARIC OXYGEN THERAPY CHAMBER

A pressurized chamber in which a patient receives pure oxygen at more than normal atmospheric pressure at sea level.

IATROGENIC

Anything caused by a medical treatment. An example is a side effect of taking a medication.

IDIOPATHIC

Arising from an unknown or obscure cause.

IMMUNOLOGY

The science that works with the structure and function and diagnosis of the immune system.

INCIDENTAL WORKED TIME

Any time in which an individual punches in early or works late according to the time clock beyond their scheduled shift and gets paid for it.

INCIDENT REPORTING

Refers to the identification of occurrences that could have led, or did lead, to an undesirable outcome.

INCLUSION CRITERIA

The factors that allow an individual to participate in a clinical trial.

INCOME STATEMENT

The income statement (also referred to as the Profit and Loss Statement or Comparative Statement of Operations) focuses on financial performance over a specific period of time, usually one year. It provides important information about the profitability of a hospital, including information on how the hospital receives its money and how the hospital spends it.

INDEPENDENT PRACTICE ASSOCIATION (IPA)

These are networks of independent physicians that contract with Managed Care Organizations (MCOs) and employers to provide services on a negotiated per capita rate, flat retainer fee, or negotiated fee-for-service basis.

INDICATOR

A measurable variable (or characteristic) that can be used to determine the degree of adherence to a standard or the level of quality achieved.

INDIGENT

Patients whose gross income is below 200 percent of the current federal poverty guidelines adjusted for family size and that has no third party payment sources.

INDIGENT CARE

Care provided, at no cost, to people who do not have health insurance or are not covered by Medicare, Medicaid, or other public programs.

INDIRECT HOURS

Hours spent for training and orientation, meetings etc.

INDIVIDUAL MANDATE

The Affordable Care Act requires nearly everyone to have health insurance that meets minimum standards. In turn, everyone would be guaranteed coverage, regardless of age or preexisting conditions.

INELIGIBLE

A patient that is not covered by insurance, the insurance does not cover certain treatments, the patient's insurance has expired, and/or the hospital stay was not approved.

INFANT

A child younger than 12 months of age.

INFANT MORTALITY

The number of infants dying at age less than 12 months divided by the number of births during that 12 months.

INFECTION

The presence of and multiplication of bacteria, viruses and parasites that are not normally present within the body.

INFECTION CONTROL COMMITTEE

The hospital committee composed of infection control personnel and medical, nursing, laboratory, and administrative staff members (and occasionally others, such as dietary or housekeeping staff members) whose purpose is to oversee infection control activities.

INFECTION CONTROL DEPARTMENT

The Infection Control department is primarily responsible for conducting surveillance of hospital acquired infections and investigating and controlling outbreaks or infections among patients and health care personnel. The department calculates rates of hospital-acquired infections, collates antibiotic susceptibility data, performs analysis of aggregated infection data and provides comparative data to national benchmarks over time.

INFECTIOUS DISEASE

Physician that specializes in the diagnosis and treatment of infections due to viral, bacterial, fungal or parasitic causes; for example, Lyme disease, hepatitis and malaria.

INFLAMMATION

Pain, redness, warmth or swelling as a result of infection, irritation or injury.

INFORMATICS

Refers to the way data is processed, stored and retrieved. Within healthcare it usually includes behavioral or medical data and financial trends.

INFORMATION DESK

This hospital function is usually located in the main lobby and is staffed by volunteers. They provide general information and directions to patient rooms or hospital departments

INFORMATION GOVERNANCE

Focuses on all types of data both structured and unstructured. Its focus is on the appropriate use of data, the value of the data and interpreting the information that the data represents.

INFORMATION TECHNOLOGY (IT)

The department that provides end users with help desk support and maintains all hospital servers, switches, and other IT Devices. They ensure that downtime of any equipment is kept to a minimum. The department is responsible for the software, hardware, and support services of the hospital information management system. This support includes but is not limited to ongoing maintenance of current hardware, the evaluation and installation of new software and hardware systems, as well as clinical application, financial application, network, PC and operations support for such systems.

Informed Consent

The requirement that a patient (or resident in a skilled nursing facility) be apprised of the nature, risks, and alternatives of a medical procedure or treatment before the physician or other health care professional begins any such procedure or treatment.

Infusion Pump

An electro-mechanical device that delivers measured amounts of fluids or medications into the bloodstream over a period of time.

In-Network

Refers to the health care facilities or providers that are part of a health plan's network of providers with which it has negotiated a discount. Insured individuals typically pay less when using an in-network provider because those networks provide services at a lower cost to the insurance companies with which they have contracts.

Inpatient

An adult or pediatric patient receiving acute care through admission to the hospital for a stay of longer than 24 hours. This does not include births.

Inpatient Days

The number of adult or pediatric patients receiving care in a hospital during the reporting period. This does not include births.

Inpatient Prospective Payment System (IPPS)

A system of classification for inpatient hospital services based on principle diagnosis, secondary diagnosis, surgical procedures, age, sex and presence of complications. This classification system is used as a financing mechanism to reimburse hospital and selected other providers for services rendered. Hospitals receive a set dollar amount, determined in advance, based on the length of time patients with a given diagnosis are likely to stay in the hospital. Also called diagnosis related groups or DRGs.

Inpatient Revenue

The total billed charges for inpatient services rendered.

Inspection

An examination of the delivered material, supplies, services, and/ or equipment ordered prior to acceptance. The process is aimed at forming a judgment as to whether the delivered items are what was ordered, were properly delivered and are ready for acceptance.

INSTITUTIONAL REVIEW BOARD (IRB):

A group of researchers and members of the public that reviews studies proposed by investigators to ensure that the study is managed in a way that protects those who participate in it. Federal regulation requires that all clinical trials must be approved by the IRB prior to enrolling participants.

INSTRUMENTAL ACTIVITIES OF DAILY LIVING (IADL)

The activities that are essential during a normal day for a person to live independently in a community. These activities may include, managing money, shopping, telephone use, house-keeping, preparing meals, and taking medications correctly.

INSURANCE EXCHANGE

A state-based organization that is designed to offer enrollees different private health insurance plans. An exchange is intended to provide consumers with transparent information about plan provisions such as premium costs and covered benefits, as well as a plan's performance in encouraging wellness, managing chronic illnesses, and improving consumer satisfaction.

INSURED

The insured is the term used to designate the person who represents the family unit in relation to the insurance program. This may be the employee whose employment makes this coverage possible. This person may also be known as the enrolee, certificate holder, policyholder, or subscriber.

INSURED GROUP NAME

Name of the group or insurance company plan that insures an individual, which is usually an employer.

INSURED GROUP NUMBER

A number that an insurance company uses to identify the group under which a patient is insured.

INSURED'S NAME (BENEFICIARY)

The name of the insured person.

INTEGRATED DELIVERY SYSTEM (IDS)

An integrated delivery system (IDS) is a network of health care providers and organizations which provides or arranges to provide a coordinated continuum of services to a defined population and is willing to be held clinically and fiscally accountable for the clinical outcomes and health status of the population served. An IDS may own or could be closely aligned with an insurance product.

INTEGRATED SUPPLY CHAIN

A long term commitment between two or more hospitals that allows them to consolidate their purchases in order to achieve mutual financial and clinical benefits.

INTEGRATION

This term refers to the process of bringing parts of a related system together or combining disparate parts together.

INTENSIVE CARE UNIT (ICU)

The Intensive Care Unit (ICU) provides comprehensive and continuous care for the critically ill adult patient with complex multi-system health problems. It is staffed 24 hours a day by specially trained Registered Nurses who are certified in advanced cardiac life support. This unit contains monitoring and specialized support equipment for patients who (because of shock, trauma, or threatening conditions) require intensified, comprehensive observation and care.

INTERFACE

The point at which two independent systems meet and act on or communicate with each other. This could be between hardware devices, between software programs, between devices and programs, or between a device and a user.

INTERMEDIATE CARE NURSERY (ICN)

A nursery for growing premature and ill newborns who are not ready to be discharged home; but do not require a Newborn Intensive Care Unit (NICU) for their care.

INTERNAL MEDICINE

The branch of medicine that provides short and long term management of common and complex medical illnesses of adolescents, adults and the elderly.

INTERNATIONAL CLASSIFICATION OF DISEASES, INTERNATIONAL (ICD-10-CM)

This is a revision to the ICD-9-CM system and is used by physicians and other health care providers to classify and code all diagnoses, symptoms and procedures recorded in conjunction with hospital care in the United States. The ICD-10-CM revision includes more than 68,000 diagnostic codes, compared to 13,000 in ICD-9-CM. In addition, ICD-10-CM includes twice as many categories and introduces alphanumeric category classifications for the first time.

INTERNSHIP

After graduating from medical school, the first year of patient care training, to be followed by residency.

INTEROPERABILITY

Describes the extent to which technology systems and devices used by healthcare organizations can exchange data, and interpret that shared data for providers.

INTRA

A prefix that indicates within.

INTRACRANIAL PRESSURE (ICP)

The pressure inside the skull and thus in the brain tissue and cerebrospinal fluid (CSF).

INTRA-HOSPITAL TRANSFER

An in-hospital discharge from one level of care to another level of care, usually from intensive care to medical/surgical care.

INTRAOPERATIVE PERIOD

The period of time during a surgical operation.

INTRAVENOUS

A catheter that is inserted into a vein so that fluid, blood or medications can be received.

INTUBATION

The Insertion of a tube into the trachea (windpipe) through the nose or mouth to allow air to reach the lungs.

INVASIVE PROCEDURE

Invasion of the body by a knife, a catheter, a cannula.

INVENTORY

Goods and supplies held in stock by the hospital or health care entity.

INVENTORY CONTROL

The control of merchandise, materials, goods in process, finished goods, and supplies on hand by accounting and physical methods.

INVENTORY MANAGEMENT

The process of monitoring and controlling the goods and supplies held in the inventory to ensure appropriate service levels are maintained.

INVENTORY TURNOVER

A term used in accounting to measure of the number of times inventory is sold or used in a time period such as a year.

INVESTIGATIONAL DEVICE EXEMPTION (IDE)

The permission that is granted by the Food and Drug Administration to use a new medical device during a clinical trial.

INVESTOR OWNED HOSPITAL

A hospital operated by a for-profit corporation in which the profits go to shareholders who own the corporation. Also referred to as a proprietary hospital or a for-profit hospital.

INVITATION TO BID (ITB)

The solicitation document utilized to solicit bids in the formal, sealed bid procedure and all documents attached or incorporated by reference.

INVOICE

A list of goods or services sent to a purchaser showing information including prices, quantities and shipping charges for payment.

INVOICE DISCREPANCY

A situation created when an invoice is cleared for payment, but a reason exists within the hospitals payment system to prevent this. Reasons might include, the invoice amount would send the order over the set Not to Exceed (NTE) limit, the order is closed, etc. Discrepancies must be cleared before an invoice can be paid.

INVOICE VERIFICATION

The matching of documents created during the purchase order process, the goods receipt process, and the accounts payable process that is part of the internal controls system within the facility.

IRRIGATE

A term that means to wash out with fluid. For example wounds are often irrigated with water or saline solution.

IRRIGATION

The washing out of a cavity or wound.

JAUNDICE

A yellowing of the skin and the whiteness of the eyes with bilirubin. It is often an indicator of liver or gall bladder disease.

JOINT COMMISSION

An organization that evaluates and accredits healthcare organizations and programs in the United States. The Joint Commission is an independent, not-for-profit organization. A hospital is accredited by the Joint Commission if it meets certain quality standards. These checks are done at least every 3 years. Most hospitals take part in these accreditations.

JOINT VENTURE

A legal arrangement between two or more entities to provide service(s), product(s) or both.

JUST-IN-TIME PURCHASING/STOCKLESS PURCHASING (JIT)

A supply system organized so that the right amount of medical supplies is made available at the correct time in order to avoid the cost of maintaining a large supply inventory.

K

The chemical symbol for potassium.

KEY PERFORMANCE INDICATORS (KPIs)

Any business metric used to evaluate factors that are important to the success of the organization i.e. hospital.

LABORATORY

The physical location where tests ordered by physicians for inpatients are done on clinical specimens in order to get information about the health of a patient pertaining to the diagnosis, treatment, and prevention of disease. Testing is usually performed in hematology, chemistry, coagulation, serology, urinalysis, blood bank, microbiology and virology by skilled medical laboratory technologists and technicians. Laboratory testing is performed under the direction of a board-certified pathologist.

LABORATORY CHARGES

Charges for diagnostic and routine clinical laboratory tests.

LAB DRAW

The process of taking blood or urine for laboratory analysis.

LABOR EXPENSES

The sum of payroll expenses and employee benefits.

LAB RESULT

The result of a test performed in a medical laboratory.

LAB TURN AROUND TIME

The amount of time it takes the laboratory to process test results.

LAPAROSCOPE

A type of endoscope consisting of a tube containing a fiber-optic cable used to examine the interior of the abdomen.

LAPAROSCOPY

An operation or procedure in which the surgeon uses an instrument called a laparoscope to view the inside of the abdominal (stomach area) cavity, through a small (less than one centimeter) incision. This is minimally invasive surgery.

LATE BIDS OR QUOTATIONS

A bid or proposal received at the place specified in the solicitation after the time designated for all bids or quotations are to be received.

LAUNDRY

The department that is responsible for providing an adequate and constant supply of stain free and germ free linen to all patients receiving care.

LEAN SIX SIGMA

A managerial approach that combines Six Sigma methods and tools and lean manufacturing principles to drive out waste and unnecessary cost and thereby provide more efficient patient care. See Six Sigma.

LEAPFROG GROUP

A group of more than 160 organizations that buy healthcare and who are working to initiate breakthrough improvements in the safety, quality, and affordability of healthcare for Americans.

LEFT WITHOUT BEING SEEN (LWBS)

Any patient encounter that ended with the patient leaving the healthcare facility before being seen by a licensed physician. The most common cause is wait-time.

LENGTH OF STAY (LOS)

The period of hospitalization as measured in days billed; average length of stay is determined by discharge days divided by discharges.

LETTER OF INTENT

An interim agreement that outlines the main points of a proposed deal, or confirms that a certain course of action is going to be taken. It is not a contract but a signal of significant interest.

LICENSED BEDS

The number of facility beds licensed by the State Department of Health.

LICENSED FACILITIES

Health care locations or facilities that require licensure from the state or national government to offer health care services. They include: hospitals, hospices, nursing homes, home health agencies, etc.

LICENSE NUMBER

The number assigned by the State Department of Health to the facility.

LICENSURE

Mandatory state-imposed standards that practitioners must meet to practice in a given profession.

LIFE EXPECTANCY

The average amount of time a person will live. In medicine it is usually calculated at birth or after the diagnosis of a disease.

LIFE SAVING MEASURE

Any life saving measure that is used when a patient's life is threatened.

LIFETIME BENEFIT MAXIMUM

The total dollar amount the healthcare plan will pay for all types of medical expenses, for all benefit periods, while an individual is alive and covered under the plan.

LIQUID ASSET

Cash in banks and on hand, and other cash assets not set aside for specific purposes other than the payment of a current liability, or a readily marketable investment.

LIQUIDITY METRICS

Financial ratios that measure the ability of a corporation to meet its short-term liabilities as they come due.

LIMITATIONS

A "cap" or limit on the amount of services that may be provided. It may be the maximum cost or number of days that a service or treatment is covered.

LIFE BIRTHS

The annual number of surviving births delivered at the hospital.

LIVING WILL

A written statement that documents a person's wish that life-sustaining treatment, including artificially or technologically supplied nutrition and hydration, be withheld or withdrawn if the person is unable to make informed medical decisions and are in a terminal condition or in a permanently unconscious state. A Living Will does not affect the responsibility of health care personnel to provide comfort care to the patient. Comfort care means any measure taken to diminish pain or discomfort, but not to postpone death.

LOGISTICS

The integration of information, transportation, inventory, warehousing, material-handling, and packaging between the point of origin and the point of consumption in order to meet the requirements of healthcare personnel and their patients.

LONG-TERM ACUTE CARE HOSPITAL (LTACH)

A hospital that specializes in treating patients with serious and often complex medical conditions requiring an average length of stay of at least 25 days. LTACHs provide care for such conditions as respiratory failure, non-healing wounds and other medically complex diseases. LTACHs are either free standing or hospitals-within-hospitals.

LONG-TERM CARE (LTC)

Services needed by people to live independently in the community, such as home health and personal care, as well as services provided in institutional settings such as skilled nursing facilities. Medicaid is the primary payer for long-term care.

LONG TERM CARE POLICY

An insurance policy that covers specified services for a specified period of time. Covered services often include nursing care, home health care services, and custodial care. Medicare does not cover most long-term care services but Medicaid does for people who qualify based on income.

LOW BIRTH WEIGHT (LBW)

A baby born weighing less than 5 1/2 pounds (2,500 grams) and more than 3.3 pounds, (1,500 grams).

LOWEST QUALIFIED PRICE

The basis for awarding contracts for commodities and or services among responsive and qualified vendors.

LUMBAR PUNCTURE (LP)

A diagnostic procedure to collect a sample of spinal fluid for analysis. It is also known as a "spinal tap." This test involves inserting a hollow needle in between the vertebrae of the lower back to collect a sample of cerebrospinal fluid.

MACRO

A prefix meaning large or long.

MAGNET HOSPITAL STATUS

An award given by the American Nurses Credentialing Center (ANCC) to hospitals that satisfy a set of criteria designed to measure the strength and quality of their nursing.

MAGNETIC RESONANCE IMAGING (MRI)

A specialized medical device that employs a magnetic field to produce high-quality images of the inside of the human body. The images that are produced are the visual equivalent of a slice of the anatomy.

MAINTENANCE

The effort used to maintain assets in a fit condition so they can perform their work. Routine maintenance is a preventive activity.

MALIGNANT TUMOR

Cancerous cells that penetrate the tissues or organs in which it originated as well as moves to other sites.

MALPRACTICE

Failure of an individual to provide acceptable and ordinary skill in their profession. Also called professional misconduct.

MALPRACTICE INSURANCE

Coverage for medical professionals which pays the costs of legal fees and/or any damages assessed by the court in a lawsuit brought against a professional who has been charged with negligence.

MAMMOGRAPHY

A diagnostic procedure to detect breast tumors through the use of X-rays.

MANAGED CARE ORGANIZATION (MCO)

A healthcare delivery system that attempts to manage the quality and cost of medical services that individuals receive. They contract with health care providers and medical facilities to provide care for members at a reduced cost. These providers make up the plan's network. The amount of care the plan will pay depends on the plans rules.

There are three types of managed care plans:

- Health Maintenance Organizations (HMO) usually only pay for care within the network. Individuals must choose a primary care physician who coordinates their patient care.

- Preferred Provider Organizations (PPO) usually pay more if the individual gets care within the network. They will pay part of the cost if the individual goes outside the network.

- Point of Service (POS) plans let an individual choose between an HMO or a PPO each time they need care.

MANDATE
Law requiring that a health plan or insurance carrier must offer a particular procedure or type of coverage.

MANDATORY REPORTING
The legal requirement that physicians and other professionals must follow to report suspected incidents of abuse and neglect. The term may also refer to reporting of defective equipment to the US Food and Drug Administration.

MARK-UP
The amount added to the cost of an item to determine the price charged to a patient or consumer.

MARKET SEGMENTATION
The process of dividing the market into distinct customer components or segments.

MARKETING DEPARTMENT
Develops and implements the hospital's marketing plan to promote hospital services.

MATERIALS MANAGEMENT
The department responsible for the procurement, processing and distribution of supplies, equipment and services through the various departments within the hospital. Also called Strategic Procurement or Strategic Sourcing.

MATERNAL & FETAL MEDICINE
The branch of medicine that provides specialized care to pregnant women and their fetuses. Also called Perinatology.

MEANINGFUL USE
The specific criteria that was developed by the Centers for Medicare & Medicaid Services (CMS) that demonstrate that the electronic health record technology utilized by a healthcare provider is connected in a way that allows for the electronic exchange of health information in accordance with all applicable laws and standards.

MEASUREMENT

The process of collecting data to assess performance conducted at a single point in time or repeated over time.

MEDICAID

Federal government healthcare assistance provided to states. The program covers individuals who are indigent and lack the financial means to pay their healthcare and hospitalization bills. The individuals who qualify for this program can vary from state to state.

MEDICAL BILLING FRAUD

When a provider improperly bills patients for services that never occurred, when they bill patients for a higher level of a service than they provided or simply provide unnecessary services.

MEDICAL BILLING SOFTWARE

Any software that is designed to process, submit and follow up on medical claims.

MEDICAL DEVICE

An apparatus, instrument, implant, in vitro reagent or other unit that operates by physical, mechanical or thermal means within the body to prevent, diagnose or treat diseases or other conditions.

MEDICAL DEVICE TECHNOLOGIES

Anything that aids a medical device to perform the diagnosis, monitoring, or treatment of a medical condition. Examples include electromechanical, medical and therapeutic radiation, software solutions, imaging, biological devices, diagnostic equipment, respiratory, in vitro diagnostics and dental.

MEDICAL DOCTOR (MD)

Medical doctor or doctor of medicine is one of two doctoral degrees that are granted by USA medical schools. The other is the Doctor of Osteopathy (DO).

MEDICAL ERROR

Any error or omission in the medical care provided to an individual. Medical errors can occur in the diagnosis, treatment or monitoring of patients or with the equipment used.

MEDICAL EXECUTIVE COMMITTEE (MEC)

The primary governance committee for the independent medical staff that makes key leadership decisions related to medical staff policies, procedures, and rules, with an emphasis on quality control and quality improvement initiatives. They are also responsible for adopting and implementing medical staff policies and procedures, and creating medical staff appointment and reappointment criteria.

MEDICAL HOME

A patient-centered health care philosophy that is intended to increase primary care excellence. The focal point through which all individuals regardless of age, sex, race, or socioeconomic status receive their acute, chronic and preventive medical care services that are accessible, accountable, comprehensive, compassionate, coordinated, integrated, patient/family-centered, safe, scientifically valid and satisfying to both patients and physicians.

MEDICAL INTENSIVE CARE UNIT (MICU)

Intensive care unit for patients with complex and multi-system disorders.

MEDICAL LIBRARY

The department that houses all of the books and journals covering all medical specialties, as well as nursing and administration. The collection is cataloged according to the National Library of Medicine Classification System.

MEDICALLY NECESSARY

Health care services or supplies needed to prevent, diagnose or treat an illness, injury, condition, disease or its symptoms and that meets accepted standards of medicine.

MEDICAL RECORD

A patient's file containing sufficient information to clearly identify the patient, to justify the patient's diagnosis, and treatment and to accurately document the results. The record also serves as a basis for planning and the continuity of patient care, and provides a means of communication among physicians and any other professionals involved in the patient's care. The record also serves as a basis for review, study, evaluations on services, and protecting the legal interests of the patient, hospital, and responsible practitioner.

MEDICAL RECORD NUMBER

This is the number assigned to the patient during their first visit to the hospital and it never changes. This is the patient's unique Hospital ID number and is used to access their personal information. It is also used for all subsequent admissions to the hospital

MEDICAL RECORDS DEPARTMENT

The department that maintains all records and documents related to patient care to meet medical, administrative, legal, ethical, regulatory, and institutional requirements of a hospital. A written medical record must be maintained on every person who is admitted or treated at the hospital. All medical records are kept confidential and in accordance with HIPAA rules and regulations.

MEDICAL RESEARCH

Any research activity performed in concert with clinical care.

MEDICAL SERVICES

Any service that pertains to medical care and that is performed for patients under the direction of a physician and other professional or technical personnel.

MEDICAL SUPPLY COSTS PER CASE

The average costs per case. It includes the cost of all disposable supplies and implants. Tracking this metric allows hospitals to monitor medical costs per specialty and by surgeon.

MEDICAL STAFF

The organized body of licensed physicians and other licensed individuals permitted by law and by the hospital to provide patient care services independently in the hospital. Appointments to the medical staff usually fall into one of the following categories:

- Attending: Those physicians that have full admitting privileges commensurate with their ability and qualifications. These physicians also serve on committees and are often department directors.

- Associate: New applicants to the medical staff. They are often appointed as associate members for 2-4 years then they become attending.

- Courtesy: Physicians and other licensed individuals who meet qualifications for appointment to the medical staff but who admit patients to the hospital only occasionally or act only as consultants and who are ineligible to participate in medical staff activities.

- Consulting: Physicians that are not member of the attending medical staff but who have been asked to provide their clinical opinion.

- House Staff: Licensed physicians that are employed by the hospital and that provide care to inpatients.

MEDICAL STAFF-ACTIVE

Physicians and other licensed individuals on the medical staff who regularly provide medical services within the hospital and who participate in all medical staff activities.

MEDICAL STAFF BYLAWS

The articles and amendments that constitute the basic governing documents of the Medical Staff.

MEDICAL STAFF RULES & REGULATIONS

The compendium of rules and regulations promulgated by the medical staff and approved by the governing board to govern specific administrative and patient care issues that arise at the hospital.

MEDICAL STAFF PRIVILEGES

Prerogatives of individuals to provide medical or other patient care services within the hospital, within well-defined limits, based on the individual's professional license, experience, competence, ability and judgment. Also referred to as clinical privileges, medical staff privileges or privileges.

MEDICAL SUPPLY COSTS PER CASE

The average costs per case. It includes the cost of all disposable supplies and implants. Tracking this metric allows hospitals to monitor medical costs per specialty and by surgeon.

MEDICAL TOURISM

When an individual travels outside the country of their residence for the purpose of receiving medical care.

MEDICAL TRANSCRIPTION

The process of converting dictated or handwritten instructions, observations, and documentation into digital text formats.

MEDICALLY NECESSARY

A term used to describe the supplies and services provided to diagnose and treat a medical condition in accordance with the standards of good medical practice and the medical community.

MEDICAL/SURGICAL

Beds not designated as perinatal, pediatric, ICU, CCU, other ICUs, burn center, intermediate care nursery and acute rehabilitation.

MEDICAL/SURGICAL UNIT

A unit that provides care for adult patients admitted with a medical condition or post-surgical condition.

MEDICARE (TITLE XVII)

A federal third-party reimbursement program administered by the Social Security Administration that underwrites the medical costs of persons age 65 and over and some qualified persons under age 65.

MEDICARE ADMINISTRATIVE CONTRACTOR (MAC)

Contractors with the federal government that process Medicare claims.

MEDICARE ADVANTAGE (MA) PLANS

A program created by the Balanced Budget Act of 1997 as Medicare + Choice and given a new name under the Medicare Prescription Drug Improvement and Modernization Act of 2003. Beneficiaries have the choice during an open season each year to enroll in a Medicare Advantage plan or to remain in traditional Medicare. Medicare Advantage plans may include coordinated care plans (HMOs, PPOs or plans offered by provider-sponsored organizations); private fee-for-service plans; or high-deductible plans with medical savings accounts.

MEDICARE ASSIGNMENT

A provider who will not bill a patient for more than the rates Medicare defines as reasonable and customary.

MEDICARE COST REPORT

An annual report required of institutions participating in the Medicare program that records each institution's total cost and charges associated with providing services to all patients, the portion of those costs and charges allocated to Medicare patients, and the Medicare payments received.

MEDICARE PART A

The hospital insurance portion of Medicare that pays for inpatient hospital care.

MEDICARE, PART B

Voluntary portion of Medicare that covers things like physicians' services and hospital out-patient services. Participants may enroll on a monthly premium basis.

MEDICARE RIGHTS FORM

This document informs Medicare patients of their rights to services and discharge. It must be signed and dated by all Medicare patients.

MEDICARE SELECT

A Medicare supplement that uses a preferred provider organization (PPO) to supplement Medicare Part B coverage.

MEDICARE SEVERITY DRG SYSTEM (MS-DRG)

This is the most widely used DRG system because it governs Medicare patients. One MS-DRG is assigned for each inpatient stay and they are assigned using the principal diagnosis and additional diagnoses, the principal procedure and additional procedures, sex and discharge status.

MEDICARE SHARED SAVINGS PROGRAM

A program that allows accountable care organizations (ACOs) to share a percentage of any savings should the actual per capita expenditures of their assigned Medicare beneficiaries fall below their specified benchmark amount.

MEDICARE SUPPLEMENT

A private medical expense insurance policy that provides reimbursement for out-of-pocket expenses, such as deductibles and coinsurance payments, or benefits for some medical expenses specifically excluded from Medicare coverage.

MEDICATION ERROR

An unintentional error in the prescribing, dispensing, administration or monitoring of a medicine that may cause or lead to inappropriate medication use or patient harm while the medication is in the control of the health care professional, patient, or consumer.

MEDICATION RECONCILIATION

A formal process of obtaining a complete and accurate list of each patient's current home medications – including name, dosage, frequency, and route – and comparing the physician's admission, transfer, and/or discharge orders to that list. Discrepancies are brought to the attention of the prescriber and, if required, changes are made to the orders.

MEDIGAP POLICY

A Medicare supplemental insurance policy that is sold by a private insurance company to fill gaps in basic Medicare coverage.

MEDLINE

The bibliographic database of the National Library of Medicine that covers medicine, nursing, dentistry, the healthcare system and others.

MEMBER

The person enrolled in a health plan.

MENTAL HEALTH/PSYCHIATRY

A physician that specializes in the diagnosis, treatment and prevention of mental and emotional disorders.

META-ANALYSIS

A statistical process that combines the findings from several different research studies.

METRICS

A method for measuring or evaluating something. Hospitals measure financial, operational, human capital, satisfaction, clinical quality and other metrics.

mHEALTH

An abbreviation for mobile health, the term for all mobile devices and apps that allow patients and providers to monitor health information. It is a rapidly growing area for both patients and providers.

MICRO

A prefix meaning small.

MICROBIOLOGY TESTING

Refers to the area of clinical pathology related to the analysis of micro-organisms such as bacteria, fungi and parasites.

MICROSURGERY

Surgery performed through a microscope using delicate instruments and precise techniques.

MILESTONE

A significant event or stage. This is a typical term used with hospital projects or initiatives.

MINIMALLY INVASIVE SURGERY

Surgery involving as few small cuts into the skin as possible. It results in decreased post-operative pain, less blood loss and a faster recovery. It's done in orthopedic, OB/GYN, neurology and general procedures.

MODIFIED RELEASE MEDICINES

Medications that are slowly released into the body to reduce how fast the body absorbs the medicine. Also called extended-release, prolonged release, controlled-release, controlled delivery, slow release and sustained-release medicines.

MORBIDITY RATE

The rate of disease, illness or accidents among a patient population.

MORGUE

The area of the hospital where an autopsy can be performed and that stores the dead.

MORTALITY RATE

The death rate amongst a patient population.

MOST FAVORED NATION CLAUSE

A contractual agreement between a supplier and a customer that requires the supplier to sell to the customer on pricing terms that are at least as favorable as the pricing terms on which that supplier sells to its other customers. In healthcare, these clauses are sometimes included in contracts between health plans and providers, but have been outlawed in a number of states.

MULTI-HOSPITAL SYSTEM

Two or more hospitals owned, leased, contract managed, or sponsored by a central organization; they can be either not-for-profit or for-profit (investor-owned).

NA

The chemical symbol for sodium.

NARCOTIC

A substance that can suppress the perception of pain by reducing the number of pain signals sent by the nervous system. Also called an Opioid or Opiate.

NASOGASTRIC TUBE (NG TUBE)

A narrow, flexible tube that is inserted through the nostril, down the esophagus, and into the stomach. It is used to give food or to remove air or fluid from the stomach.

NATIONAL PATIENT SAFETY GOALS (NPSG)

A program started by the Joint Commission in 2002. They were established to help accredited organizations address specific areas of concern in regard to patient safety issues in a wide variety of health care settings. Each year an advisory group called the Patient Safety Advisory Group meets and advises The Joint Commission on how to address those issues. The Joint Commission also determines whether a goal is applicable to a specific accreditation program and, if so, tailors the goal to be program-specific.

NATIONAL PRACTITIONER DATABANK (NPPB)

An alert or flagging system created to provide a more comprehensive review of professional credentials. It assists state licensing boards, hospitals and other healthcare entities in conducting intensive independent reviews of the qualifications of the healthcare practitioner they seek to license or to grant clinical privileges to. Information reported to the national practitioner data bank is confidential except to those legally allowed to access it.

NATIONAL PROVIDER IDENTIFIER (NPI):

A unique 10-digit identification number assigned to healthcare providers in the U.S. by CMS.

NATIONAL TIME OUT DAY

An event that occurs on June 10th of every year designed to draw attention to the need for everyone on the surgical team to pause before the surgical procedure begins in order to make sure they are operating on the right patient, the right site and they are performing the right procedure.

NEAR MISS

An event or situation that did not produce patient injury but could have, only because of chance. Also referred to as a "close call."

NEONATAL

The part of an infant's life from the hour of birth through the first 28 days.

NEONATOLOGY

The specialized care and treatment of a newborn up to six weeks of age.

NEONATOLOGY- NEONATAL-PERINATAL MEDICINE

The field of medicine that provides care and treatment of infant up to six weeks of age. Neonatologists specialize in the care of premature infants and newborns with illnesses.

NEGOTIATION

The process of reaching agreement through discussion and compromise.

NEONATAL ICU (NICU)

A hospital unit which is dedicated to the care of infants that are born prematurely or with critical illnesses. This unit is staffed with specially trained nursing personnel and contains monitoring and specialized support equipment for infants who require intensified, comprehensive observation, and care.

NEONATAL INTERMEDIATE CARE

A unit that must be separate from the normal newborn nursery and that provides intermediate and/or recovery care and some specialized services.

NEPHROLOGY

The branch of medicine that is concerned with the kidneys: It's function, problems, treatment and renal replacement i.e. dialysis and kidney transplantation.

NET INCOME (LOSS)

The mathematical difference between total operating revenue and total operating expenses.

NET INCOME FROM OPERATIONS

Total Operating Revenue minus Total Operating Expenses.

NET PATIENT SERVICE REVENUE

Inpatient and outpatient revenue for all patient care services less deductions from revenue.

NET MARGIN

Revenues in excess of operating expenses generated from patient service activities.

NETWORK

A group of providers typically linked through contractual arrangements, which provide a defined set of benefits.

NETWORK PROVIDER

Providers or health care facilities that are part of a health plan's network with which it has negotiated a discount. Insured individuals usually pay less when using a network provider.

NEUROLOGICAL ICU (NICU)

The specialty care unit that provides brain and spinal cord monitoring and treatments that are specific for the neurological patient such as continuous EEG monitoring, intra-cranial pressure (ICP) monitoring and spinal cord stabilization. May also be called Neuroscience Critical Care Unit.

NEUROLOGY

The diagnosis and treatment of the nervous system and brain. It also includes strokes and seizures.

NEURORADIOLOGY

The area within radiology that specializes in the use of radioactive substances, x-rays and scanning devices for the diagnosis and treatment of diseases of the brain, spine and nervous system.

NEUROSURGICAL

Surgery of the nervous system.

NEVER EVENT

When surgery is done on the wrong patient or wrong body part it is called a "never event" because it's never supposed to happen.

NEWBORN (NB)

An infant from birth through the first 28 days of life.

NEW TECHNOLOGY COMMITTEE

A multi-disciplinary committee that establishes the process by which new clinical products are introduced to the hospital and that provides a mechanism for existing products to be reviewed and analyzed. May also be called a Product Evaluation Committee or Value Analysis Committee.

NON-COVERED CHARGES

Charges for medical services denied or excluded by an insurance company. A patient is billed for these charges.

NON-COVERED DAYS

Days of patient care not covered by the primary payer.

NONINVASIVE

Anything that does not enter the body through the skin or an opening (mouth, nose, anus, etc.).

NONINVASIVE PROCEDURE

Treatment that does not require the clinician to use an instrument to enter the body or puncture the skin.

Non-Chargeable Items

A supply item that is not charged to the patient.

Non-File Item

A supply item that is not listed within the purchasing systems' file of available supplies for ordering.

Non-MD Employees

The number of full-time employees that are not physicians.

Non-Participating Provider

A doctor, hospital or other healthcare provider that is not part of an insurance plan's doctor or hospital network. Usually patients must pay their own healthcare costs to see a non-participating provider.

Non-Productive Hours

Non-worked hours that are paid. Examples are sick time, holiday time, personal leave, jury duty, bereavement etc.

Non-Stock item

A supply item that is not kept on hand and is only ordered when required.

Nosocomial

Relating to a hospital, especially a new disorder acquired during treatment in a hospital.

Nosocomial Infection

An infection or disease acquired in a hospital or other health care facility.

Not-for-Profit (NFP) Hospital

A hospital with a tax exemption status due to its classification as a charitable organization. The exemption, which is regulated by the IRS, allows the hospital to forego tax payment in a number of areas, the most visible of which are tax on net income, payroll and property; in return, the hospital must meet various requirements outlined by the IRS. Typically, a not-for-profit hospital is run by a board of trustees, is exempt from federal and state taxes and uses its profits to cover capital expenses and future operating costs.

Not Enabled

A supplier who is not an approved vendor of the hospital.

NOTIFICATION OF PRIVACY PRACTICES (NPP)

This form describes how the patients' medical information may be used and disclosed, and how patients can gain access to their information. This form must be signed and dated by the patient and then entered into the patients' medical record. This is part of the HIPPA Act.

NUCLEAR MEDICINE DEPARTMENT

Provides medical imaging services using radioactive isotopes to diagnose and treat disease. Nuclear Medicine services are provided through Positron Emission Tomography (PET) and Positron Emission Tomography/Computed Tomography (PET/CT) units. PET technology can detect disease processes early -- often before symptoms appear -- giving physicians a lead in treating cancer, heart disease and other medical conditions.

NUCLEAR PHARMACY

A pharmacy that is involved with the preparation of radioactive materials to improve and promote health through the safe and effective use of radioactive drugs to diagnose and treat specific disease states.

NURSE

An individual that is trained to provide care for the injured, sick, or aged.

NURSERY

A hospital unit for normal newborns.

NURSING LEVELS OF EDUCATION

The levels of education established for nursing are:

- **VOCATIONAL/LPN**
  Requires one year of formal nursing training at a vocational or technical school.

- **DIPLOMA/RN**
  Requires two-to-three years of education at a hospital school for nursing.

- **ASSOCIATE DEGREE/ASN OR AND**
  Requires two years of education at a college or university.

- **BACCALAUREATE DEGREE/BSN**
  Requires four academic years of education at a college or university

- **MASTER'S DEGREE/MSN**
  Requires completion of at least one year of prescribed study beyond the baccalaureate degree.

NURSING ROUNDS

Rounds are informal meetings of caregivers, usually held at or near the patient care area. Nursing rounds are intended specifically for communication among nurses. These usually occur at the beginning of every shift and focus on each patient and their plan of care.

NURSING SERVICES

Encompasses all activities related to nursing care performed by nurses and other professional and technical personnel.

NUTRITION SERVICES

Trained dieticians and nutritionists provide specialist advice on diet for hospital patients and outpatient clinics, forming part of a multidisciplinary team. They also provide group education to patients with diabetes, heart disease and osteoarthritis, and work closely with weight management groups.

OBESITY CLINIC

Out-patient services that provide treatment of patients with abnormal amounts of fat.

OBSOLESCENCE

The loss in usefulness of an asset.

OBSTETRICS & GYNECOLOGY (OB/GYN)

The branch of medicine that specializes in the medical and surgical care of the female reproductive system and associated disorders. The OB is an abbreviation for obstetrics or for an obstetrician, a physician who delivers babies. GYN is an abbreviation for gynecology or for a gynecologist, a physician who specializes in treating diseases of the female reproductive organs.

OBSTETRICS CLINIC

Outpatient services provided to the mother and fetus throughout pregnancy, childbirth and the immediate postpartum period.

OCCUPANCY EXPENSE

Expense relating to the use of the hospital. Examples are: rent, heat, light, depreciation, upkeep, and general care of the facility.

OCCUPANCY RATE

The percentage of facility beds occupied during the reporting period.

OCCUPATIONAL SAFETY AND HEALTH ADMINISTRATION (OSHA)

A federal organization that ensures safe and healthy working conditions for Americans by enforcing standards and by providing workplace safety training. They are a part of the Department of Labor.

OCCUPATIONAL THERAPY (OT) DEPARTMENT

Helps people who are physically or mentally impaired, including temporary disability after medical treatment. They practice in the fields of both healthcare and social care. The aim of occupational therapy is to restore physical and mental functioning to help people participate in life to the fullest. Occupational therapy assessments often guide hospital discharge planning, with the majority of patients given a home assessment to understand their support needs. Staff also arrange the provision of essential equipment and adaptations that are essential for discharge from the hospital.

OFF-HOURS SURGERY

This Operating Room key performance indicator measures the volume or percentage of surgery that is performed outside of the scheduled OR hours such as during evenings, nights, weekends and holidays. Off-hours surgery may result from emergency cases or when scheduled cases exceed their scheduled time.

OFFICE OF INSPECTOR GENERAL (OIG)

The organization responsible for establishing guidelines and investigating fraud and misinformation within the healthcare industry. The OIG is part of the Department of Health and Human Services.

ON CALL (STANDBY)

Pay that is made to an employee for being available to come into work if needed.

ONCOLOGY

The medical specialty that is devoted to cancer. Clinical oncology consists of three primary disciplines:

- Medical Oncology: The treatment of cancer with medicine, including chemotherapy.

- Surgical Oncology: The surgical aspects of cancer including biopsy and staging, and surgical resection (of tumors)

- Radiation Oncology: The treatment of cancer with therapeutic radiation.

ON-HAND INVENTORY

Supplies currently in stock and available for use.

ON-SERVICE

A period of time assigned to an attending physician when he/she is responsible and accountable for the day-to-day care of patients in his/her particular unit. A service rotation can consist of several days, or several weeks, depending on the specialty.

OPEN ACCESS

Health plan flexibility to obtain medical services from a specialist (within the plan) without referral from a primary care physician.

OPEN SURGICAL TECHNIQUE

Describes the method of performing an operation, where the surgeon makes a cut in the body.

OPERATING BUDGET

A budget covering on-going revenues and expenses.

OPERATING COST (OR EXPENSE)

An expense incurred in conducting the ordinary major activities of a hospital or business, usually excluding "non-operating" expense or income deductions.

OPERATING INCOME (OR PROFIT)

The excess of the revenues of a hospital or business over the expenses pertaining thereto, excluding income and expense derived from sources other than its regular activities.

OPERATING MARGIN

This is the most commonly used measure of a hospital's financial performance. It compares a hospital's total operating revenue against its total operating expenses, often referred to as net from operations and is calculated as follows:

Operating Margin Formula: (Total Operating Revenue – Total Operating Expenses) / Total Operating Revenue

OPERATING REVENUE

Revenue directly related to the rendering of patient care services.

OPERATING ROOM (OR)

This usually refers to a suite of rooms in a hospital or surgery center in which patients are prepared for surgery and undergo various types of surgical procedures.

OPERATING ROOM BLOCK UTILIZATION

Measured by surgeon or service. Typically, a surgeon that has a busy practice and does hip and knee replacements blocks an OR for "x" number of cases per day for "x" number of cases per week. Their block of time includes the turnaround time to get the OR ready for the next case. When this is taken into account the metric used is adjusted utilization = the total block minutes utilized + the turnaround time divided by the total block minutes available.

OPERATING ROOM OPEN TIME

The time that is available to anyone and it can be booked in advance. This is usually for surgeons that don't have a block of time reserved each week. Urgent time is the time that is available 24 hours before. This allows cases to be scheduled that need to be performed urgently but are not emergencies. Many general surgeries are examples of urgent times.

OPERATING ROOM USE

This Operating Room key performance indicator measures the percentage of OR time used compared to what was budgeted.

OPERATING ROOM UTILIZATION BY DAY OF WEEK

This Operating Room key performance indicator measures total OR utilization for each day of the week. The goal is to have an even level of usage each day to prevent large open periods. In most hospitals the goal is to have each OR in use 75-80% of the time. This allows the OR scheduler to add emergency cases as required.

OPIATE

A substance that can suppress the perception of pain by reducing the number of pain signals sent by the nervous system. Also called a Narcotic or Opioid.

OPIOID

A substance that can suppress the perception of pain by reducing the number of pain signals sent by the nervous system. Also called a Narcotic or Opiate.

OPHTHALMOLOGICAL SERVICES

Services of the eye including medical, surgical and optical care.

OPHTHALMOLOGIC SURGERY

Surgery involving the eye. Common surgeries include cataract removal, treatments for glaucoma, macular degeneration and retinal detachment, radial keratotomy (cornea repair) and vitreous replacement. Ophthalmologic surgeons also perform pediatric surgeries, including opening blocked tear ducts, correcting droopy eyelids and eye muscle repair. Many eye surgeries are handled as out-patient surgeries.

OPTIMIZATION

A term that is often used following an IT implementation. It refers to the phase where the IT system goes from being operational in terms of workflow to functioning at its peak capacity for optimal performance.

ORIGINAL COST

The price for an item.

ORTHOPEDIC

The treatment of deformities, diseases and injuries of the bones, joints and muscles.

OSTEOPATHIC

A specific type of medicine whose theory is that disturbances in the musculoskeletal system affect other body parts and functions, resulting in many disorders that can be corrected by various manipulative techniques along with conventional medical, surgical, pharmacological, and other therapeutic procedures.

OTHER OPERATING REVENUE

Includes revenue from non-patient care services to patients and sales and activities to persons other than patients. Examples include non-patient sales, gift shop and parking garage.

OTOLARYNGOLIC SERVICES

Services that relate to the medical and surgical treatment of the head and neck which includes the ears, nose and throat (ENT).

OUT-OF-STOCK

A term that is used for a supply item that is temporarily not available. Also called a Stock Out.

OUTCOMES

Measures of the effectiveness of particular kinds of medical treatment i.e. the end result of medical care, as indicated by recovery, disability, functional status, mortality, morbidity, or patient satisfaction.

OUTCOMES MEASUREMENT

The process of systematically tracking a patient's clinical treatment and responses to that treatment using quality indicators, such as mortality, morbidity, disability, functional status, recovery, and patient satisfaction.

OUTCOMES RESEARCH

Research on patient outcomes that result from specific health and medical interventions.

OUTSOURCING

A process by which an organization contracts out a business process to an independent organization to perform activities previously performed by internal staff.

OUTLIER

Patients that have longer than average lengths of stay or unusually high costs.

OUT-OF-BOX FAILURES

A designation given to products which are not functional when delivered. Also called Dead on Arrival.

OUT-OF-NETWORK-OUT OF PLAN

Refers to physicians, hospitals or other health care providers who do not participate in an insurance plan (usually an HMO or PPO). Depending on an individual's health insurance plan, expenses incurred by services provided by out-of-plan health professionals are usually not covered by an individual's insurance company and therefore must be paid out-of-pocket by the individual.

OUT-OF-POCKET COSTS

The amount of money that an individual must pay for his or her healthcare, including: deductibles, co-pays, payments for services that are not covered, and/or health insurance premiums that are not paid by his or her employer.

OUT OF POCKET MAXIMUM

The maximum amount an individual pays during a policy period (usually a calendar year) before their health insurance begins to pay 100% of the allowed amount.

OUTPATIENT

A patient who receives medical treatment without the requirement of being admitted as an inpatient to a hospital.

OUTPATIENT CLINIC

Provides outpatients with the convenience of meeting with specialties such as: Urology, OB/GYN, Cardiology, Cardiovascular Surgery, Neurosurgery, Ear/Nose/Throat (ENT), Podiatry, and Oncology. Many of the procedures and tests ordered by the specialists can also be performed at an outpatient clinic.

OUTPATIENT DIALYSIS CENTER

A facility that offers newly diagnosed patients with kidney failure and maintenance for new patients with chronic kidney failure. Services provided include hemodialysis and peritoneal dialysis.

OUTPATIENT GROSS REVENUE %

The percentage of billings for patients receiving care for less than 24 hours.

OUTPATIENT HOSPITAL CARE

Medical or surgical care received from a hospital when a physician hasn't written an order to admit an individual to the hospital as an inpatient. Outpatient hospital care may include emergency department services, observation services, outpatient surgery, lab tests etc.

OUTPATIENT PROSPECTIVE PAYMENT SYSTEM (OPPS)

The system of payment used by Medicare to pay outpatient departments of hospitals and other outpatient facilities. The specific amount that is paid is determined by the ambulatory payment classification (APC).

OUTPATIENT SURGERY

Surgery that does not require an overnight hospital stay; also called ambulatory surgery or same-day surgery.

OUTPATIENT VISITS

Visits by people to a clinic or hospital to receive a medical diagnosis or treatment but without occupying a hospital bed for a specified minimum stay. Included are emergency room visits, outpatient clinic visits, referred ancillary service visits, home health care contacts, and day care days, where the outpatient is treated and released the same day. Also included are outpatient ambulatory surgery visits, renal dialysis visits, observation care visits, psychiatric visits, chemical dependency visits, hospice outpatient visits, and adult day health care visits.

Outpatient Visits per Day

Average number of outpatient visits per day for the reporting period. Calculated by dividing the number of outpatient visits by the number of days in the reporting period.

Outsourcing

The process of contracting out a business process or service to an independent organization that can perform the function at less cost, when sufficient internal resources are not available or where the business process or service can be performed better than using internal resources.

Outstanding

Uncollected or unpaid debt.

Overhead

A general name for all costs of materials and services that is not directly added or identifiable with a hospital or service after being provided.

Over-the-Counter

A term that describes drugs that can be purchased without a prescription.

Paid Hours

Productive hours plus non-productive hours. All hours that employees are compensated for.

Paid to Provider

The amount an insurance company pays directly to a medical provider for services rendered.

Paid To You

The amount the insurance company pays the patient or guarantor.

Pain Management

The control of pain or discomfort though medication, stress reduction, exercise, relaxation techniques, massage cold, heat etc.

Pain Medicine

The area within the field of medicine that is concerned with the prevention of pain, and the evaluation, treatment, and rehabilitation of persons in pain.

Palliative Care

Care or treatment provided to release pain and improve the quality of life for patients with serious or life threatening injuries.

PARTICIPATING PROVIDER

A doctor or hospital that agrees to accept an insurance payment for covered services as payment in full, minus the patient's deductible, co-pay and coinsurance amount.

PATHOLOGY

The study of the origin, nature, and course of diseases.

PATIENT

An individual that seeks or receives medical care.

PATIENT ACCOUNTS

The department responsible for the assessment and billing of patients and external agencies, debt collection and compliance with Health Act provisions relating to billing. A key function is the collation and submission of claims to health insurers.

PATIENT ADVOCATE

A person whose job is to speak on a patient's behalf and help patients get any information or services they need.

PATIENT AMOUNT DUE

The amount charged by a doctor or hospital for which the patient is responsible to pay.

PATIENT BILL OF RIGHTS

Outlines the basic rights of each patient in a healthcare facility.

PATIENT CARE SERVICES REVENUE

The hospital's full established charges for services rendered to patients, regardless of amounts actually paid to the hospital by or on behalf of patients.

PATIENT CARE TEAM

A multidisciplinary team organized under the leadership of a physician, with each member of the team having specific individual responsibilities that contribute to the care of the patient.

PATIENT CENTERED MEDICAL HOME (PCMH)

The patient centered medical home is not a physical place but rather a method that delivers the core functions of primary health care. It has the following components: it's patient-focused, comprehensive, coordinated, accessible and focused on quality and safety.

PATIENT CHARGE LABEL

A bar-coded supply item label that is transferred from the supply item to the patient's charge when the item is used.

PATIENT DAYS

The total number of inpatient days (excluding newborns) for the reporting period.

PATIENT ENGAGEMENT

The process by which healthcare providers ensure that patients are involved and included in their own care processes.

PATIENT EXPERIENCE

A measurement that obtains reports or ratings from patients about services received from an organization, hospital, physician, or healthcare provider. Also called patient satisfaction.

PATIENT FOCUSED CARE

The concept of patient care delivery based on the principles of work simplification, multi-skilled workers and placement of services as close to the patient as possible to achieve significant quality and efficiency improvements.

PATIENT IDENTIFICATION BRACELET

A plastic band with a patient identification label affixed to it that is worn by the patient throughout hospitalization. In the obstetrics department, a mother and the newborn would share the same identification label affixed to their ID bracelets until the baby is assigned their own medical record number.

PATIENT SAFETY

Patient freedom from accidental or preventable injuries produced by the hospital care givers.

PATIENT SATISFACTION

A measurement that obtains reports or ratings from patients about services received from an organization, hospital, physician, or healthcare provider. Also called patient experience.

PATIENT SATISFACTION SURVEY

Questionnaire used to solicit the perceptions of plan enrollees or patients regarding how a hospital, physician or healthcare organization met their medical needs and how the delivery of care was handled (e.g., waiting time, access to treatments etc.).

PATIENT TRANSPORT SERVICES

Many hospitals have a transport team available 24-7-365 that helps patients by transporting them into, around, and out of the health care organization.

PATHOLOGY

The science or the study of the origin, nature, and course of diseases. The most common types are:

- Anatomical Pathology: which is the study of the structure or functional changes in tissues or organs which cause or are caused by disease.

- Clinical Pathology: which uses laboratory methods of chemical, microscopic, and serologic examinations to detect disease.

- Surgical Pathology: is the examination of specimens of tissues removed from living patients for the purpose of diagnosis of disease and guidance in the care of patients.

PAYER

A person or organization which pays the hospital for services rendered to patients. This can be the patient and/or third parties such as Medicare, Medi-Cal, Blue Cross, managed care organizations, or other private insurance plans.

PAY FOR PERFORMANCE (P4P)

A direct financial reward model or quality bonus rewarded for meeting agreed upon goals for the delivery of healthcare services.

PAYMENT

Reimbursement a hospital receives for care provided; usually less than the standard charge and sometimes less than the cost of providing care.

PAYROLL EXPENSES

All amounts paid to employees in the form of salaries and wages.

PEDIATRIC CLINIC

Outpatient services related to the diagnosis, care and treatment of children.

PEDIATRIC ANESTHESIOLOGY

The medical specialty devoted that provides anesthesia for infants and children. They are an anesthesiologist that has completed an additional year of training in anesthesia care for infants and children.

PEDIATRIC CARDIOLOGY

The medical specialty devoted that handles the diagnosis and treatment of congenital and acquired heart disease and conditions in children, ranging from newborns to young adults.

PEDIATRIC HEMATOLOGY-ONCOLOGY

The medical specialty devoted to the treatment of blood and blood system diseases in children such as serious anemia, lymphomas, sickle cell disease and cancer.

PEDIATRIC ICU (PICU)

The area of the hospital which provides specialized nursing care of the most concentrated and exhaustive nature for children. This unit is staffed with specially trained nursing personnel and contains monitoring and specialized support equipment for patients who (because of shock, trauma, or threatening conditions) require intensified, comprehensive observation, and care.

PEDIATRIC OPHTHALMOLOGY

The medical specialty devoted to care of the eye and the treatment of diseases that affect the eyes and the vision of children.

PEDIATRIC PATIENT

Children less than 14 years of age.

PEDIATRICS

The department that provides a complete line of services such as physical, emotional and social to meet the health and developmental needs of children.

PEDIATRIC SURGERY

Surgery performed on children due to injuries, deformities or disease.

PEER REVIEW

An evaluation conducted by practicing physicians or other clinical professionals of the appropriateness, effectiveness and efficiency of medical services ordered or performed by other practicing physicians or clinical professionals. Peer review of manuscripts also occurs before publication of articles in medical journals.

PERCENT PRODUCTIVE HOURS

The number of productive hours divided by the paid hours.

PERCENTAGE OF UNPLANNED OR CLOSURES

This Operating Room key performance indicator measures the percentage of OR time lost due to unplanned closures, which often results when:

- Personnel, beds, supplies or equipment are not available.

- There is inadequate notification of OR time available as a result of it being forfeited by services or surgeons.

- Environmental factors such as an outbreak of the flu.

PER DIEM

Payment to a provider (normally an acute care facility) at an established or negotiated rate per day rather than reimbursement of all hospital charges as billed.

PERCUTANEOUS LINE/PERCUTANEOUS CENTRAL CATHETER (PICC)

A long catheter inserted into a surface vein with the catheter tip extending into a larger vein. A PICC line is usually very stable and lasts longer than a typical IV.

PERFECT ORDER

The percentage of orders delivered to the right place, with the right product, at the right time, in the right condition, in the right package, in the right quantity, with the right documentation, to the right customer, with the correct invoice.

PERPETUAL INVENTORY

An inventory management method that monitors and maintains on-hand quantities of supplies at optimal levels.

PERFORMANCE MEASURE

A measure that provides an indication (e.g., index, percentage, rate, ratio) of a healthcare organization's/or provider's ability to provide care most likely to ensure a good patient outcome.

PERINATAL

The time before and after birth. It is defined in different ways but it always starts between week 20- 28 of gestation and ends somewhere between 1-4 weeks after birth.

PERINATAL CARE

Health care services provided to mothers and newborns from pregnancy through the first month of the infant's life.

PERINATOLOGY

The branch of medicine that provides specialized care to pregnant women and their fetuses. Also called Maternal & Fetal Medicine.

PERIOPERATIVE

The time just before and/or just after surgery.it includes the time a patient goes into a facility for surgery until they are discharged.

PERSONAL CARE

Nonskilled, personal care, such as help with bathing, dressing, eating, getting in and out of bed or a chair, and using the bathroom. The Medicare home health benefit pays for these services.

PERSONAL HEALTH INFORMATION (PHI)

Usually refers to demographic information such as medical history, test and laboratory results, insurance information and other data that a healthcare professional collects to identify an individual and determine appropriate care. Also called Protected Health Information.

PERSONNEL DEPARTMENT

The department that is responsible for the recruitment of new employees and retention of current employees. The responsibilities include employee relations, benefits administration, policy implementation, staffing and knowledge of all laws & regulations pertaining to human resources. The department also acts as a liaison between administration and staff assisting in the development of appropriate programs/plans in the resolution of the everyday business and workforce challenges. Also called Human Resources Department.

PHARMACOECONOMICS

The study of the costs and the benefits of various pharmaceutical treatments.

PHARMACY

Controls the preparation, dispensing, storage, and use of drugs. It generally services inpatients, outpatients, clinic and emergency patients. The pharmacy provides a drug formulary for the hospital physicians to use as a guide. It also helps supervise any clinical trial management and drug-use review.

PHARMACY AND THERAPEUTICS (P&T) COMMITTEE

A panel composed of physicians, pharmacists and other clinicians who evaluate pharmaceuticals and therapeutic agents in order to optimize pharmaceutical utilization; this group usually approves and maintains the organization's drug formulary.

PHARMACY COMPOUNDING

The art and science of preparing personalized medications for patients.

PHOTOTHERAPY

Treatment with light for jaundice in a newborn. Often newborns are placed under a special light to help the body break down the extra bilirubin in their blood.

PHYSICAL INVENTORY

Within hospitals it is the inventory that is determined by physically viewing and counting the devices or consumables and in relevant cases by weighing or measuring amounts.

PHYSICAL LIFE

The total potential operating life of a device as compared with the useful life which may be much less because of obsolescence or because it is no longer adequate due to improvements in technology.

PHYSICAL MEDICINE AND REHABILITATION

Also known as physiatry, physical medicine and rehabilitation. This department and their physicians focus on the diagnosis and treatment of people with physical and/or cognitive impairment or disability. Physiatrists work to restore or develop a broad spectrum of functioning for people whose abilities have been limited by disease, trauma, congenital disorder or pain.

PHYSICAL THERAPY (PT) DEPARTMENT)

Physical therapy is the art and science of physical care and rehabilitation. Physical therapists provide services to individuals to develop, maintain, and restore maximum movement and functional ability throughout their life. This includes providing services in circumstances where movement and function are threatened by aging, injury, disease or environmental factors.

PHYSICIAN

A doctor of medicine or of osteopathy who is fully licensed to practice medicine.

PHYSICIAN ALIGNMENT

When the hospital and the medical staff see a mutually beneficial relationship that is symbiotic around the mission of the hospital and the goals of each party. The goals usually relate to clinical, emotional, financial and spiritual.

PHYSICIAN- ATTENDING

The physician that has a legal responsibility for the care of a patient within the hospital.

PHYSICIAN DESK REFERENCE (PDR)

A complete listing of all the drugs (primarily prescription drugs) used in diagnostic procedures in the U.S. The information provided is the same as that listed in the package insert. Drug manufacturers pay to have their drug included in the PDR so many generic medicines will not be included.

PHYSICIAN EMPLOYEES

The number of full-time hospital employed physicians.

PHYSICIAN OWNED DISTRIBUTORSHIP (POD)

A business arrangement that involves one or more physician owning a medical device distributor or company. There are a variety of business models available but typically a physician purchases a share or ownership interest of a medical device company in exchange for a cash investment in which he /she believes they will achieve a high return on their investment. Oftentimes, PODs are formed with a physician or group practice to sell and/or distribute devices to hospitals or surgical centers where the physician-investors are also performing surgical procedures that utilize the same devices distributed through their company. PODs are common with many implantable medical devices. This enables surgeons to control what medical devices they use during a procedure, and to share in the profits generated by the sale of those devices. They bill for the surgical procedure separately.

PHYSICIAN PAYMENT SUNSHINE ACT

The Sunshine Act requires companies that make drugs, medical devices and biological medicines to report payments and items of value that are given to physicians and teaching hospitals. The specifics of the law have been outlined in the Federal Register.

The law also requires that manufacturers and group purchasing organizations (GPOs) must report certain ownership interests by physicians and their immediate family.

The law states that:

- Any prescription drug or device manufacturer operating in the U.S. must report payments to physicians and teaching hospitals to the Center for Medicare and Medicaid Services (CMS). All physician disclosure data will then be posted on a public website.

- Physicians are defined as all doctors of medicine, osteopathy, podiatry, optometry, dentistry and chiropractic medicine.

- A teaching hospital is any hospital that receives payment from Medicare for graduate medical education.

- Any payments or transfers of value worth at least $10.00 and transactions of less than $10.00 if they total $100.00 or more in a calendar year must be reported.

The types of items that must be reported are honorariums, gifts, speaking fees, travel and lodging, food and beverage, entertainment, parking, etc. CMS can levy $10,000 fines on manufacturers for failing to report gifts. The penalty climbs to $100,000 when a manufacturer is found to have knowingly omitted payment information.

PHYSICIAN PREFERENCE CARDS

Basic information on physician preference information that is captured and distributed in multiple formats at each nursing station and with nursing leadership that includes contact information, rounding times and information preferred prior to rounding. For surgeons it is the foundation on which the surgical case is scheduled and the case cart is assembled. The information on the card is used to gather supplies, instrumentation, medications, equipment, and to set up the OR suite.

PHYSICIAN PREFERENCE ITEM (PPI)

Expensive products specifically requested by a physician for their use such as orthopedic implants, heart valves, bone products, balloons and wires.

PHYSICIAN SERVICES

Health care services provided or coordinated by a licensed medical physician Medical Doctor around (M.D.) or a Doctor of Osteopathic Medicine (D.O.).

PICTURE ARCHIVING AND COMMUNICATION SYSTEM - (PACS)

An information technology based storage and retrieval system for digital images.

PHYSICIAN-TEACHING

Physicians who have a primary responsibility for teaching related to graduate physicians in training or to under graduates.

PLACEBO

A substance or treatment, given as a therapeutic agent that has no medical effect. It is administered to help distinguish between real and imagined effects during experiments on patients.

PODIATRY

The care and treatment of the foot and ankle from childhood to adult including injury, disease and surgical interventions.

POINT OF CARE

Laboratory and other services provided to patients at their bedside.

POPULATION HEALTH

Usually refers to the health of an entire population of individuals within a given geography to improve their outcomes. Population health allows providers to target a specific group of patients to improve their health such as those with diabetes, COPD etc. Population health also relates to the social determinants of health and not just medical treatment.

PORTAL

This frequently applies to patient portals, which is an access interface tool whereby patients can access their medical records and log into a healthcare organization's system to make appointments, manage their prescriptions, ask questions, review test results etc.

POSITRON EMISSION TOMOGRAPHY SCANNER (PET)

A diagnostic imaging tool that uses radioactive isotopes to show details of body structures deep within a patient without interference from surrounding tissues.

POST ANESTHESIA CARE UNIT (PACU)

The unit where patients are taken to recover from surgical anesthesia and then reunited with family members.

POSTERIOR

After, in relation to time or space. The back surface of the body.

POSTNATAL CARE

Healthcare services received by a woman immediately following the delivery of her child.

POST-OPERATIVE PERIOD

The period after surgery, including the recovery time spent in the hospital and at home.

POSTPARTUM

The care of the mother following childbirth.

PRE-ADMISSION

The process of obtaining and confirming patient demographic and financial information at least twenty-four hours in advance of arrival for inpatient or outpatient services.

PRE-ADMISSION DEPOSIT

The amount a patient pays before getting medical care. Also referred to as a Pre-Payment.

PRE-ADMIT

The process of obtaining patient information and beginning the preparation of the admission forms before a patient's arrival at a hospital or out-patient facility.

PRE-AUTHORIZATION

A procedure governed by a contract used to review and assess the medical necessity and appropriateness of elective hospital admissions and non-emergency care before the services are provided. Also called prior authorization.

PRE-CERTIFICATION

A process similar to preauthorization whereby patients must check with their insurance company to see if a desired healthcare treatment or service is deemed medically necessary (and thus covered) by their insurance.

PRE-DETERMINATION

The maximum sum a healthcare plan of an insurance company will pay for certain services or treatments.

PRE-EXISTING CONDITION (PEC)

A medical condition (usually an injury, disease or disability) that a patient had before receiving coverage from an insurance company. A person might become ineligible for certain healthcare plans depending on the severity and length of their PEC.

PRE-EXISTING CONDITION EXCLUSION

A condition that denies a person certain coverage in some health insurance plans.

PRE-HOSPITAL CARE

Any care rendered by a paramedic-EMT prior to a patient arriving at a hospital.

PREDICTIVE ANALYTICS

Within healthcare predictive analytics encompasses a variety of statistical techniques to make predictions about the health of an individual or group of individuals.

PRE-EXISTING CONDITION

A health condition or medical problem that a patient already has before receiving insurance.

PREFERRED PROVIDER ORGANIZATION (PPO)

A managed care arrangement that offers enrolees a larger choice of primary care and specialty providers to choose from with fewer utilization restrictions than an HMO offers.

PREMATURE INFANT

An infant born before the 37th week of gestation.

PREMIUM

The amount that must be paid for health insurance. The employee and/or their employer usually pays it monthly, quarterly or yearly.

PRE-OPERATIVE PERIOD

The period before a surgery including the patient's pre-operative instructions and prep time before a surgery.

PRE-PAYMENT

The amount a patient pays before getting medical care; also referred to as pre-admission deposit.

PRE-QUALIFIED VENDORS

A vendor who has successfully completed the pre-qualification process.

PRE- QUALIFY

The process of ensuring that vendors selected to do business with the hospital meet established criteria before awarding business. The criteria typically include financial capability, reputation and management as a minimum.

PREMIUM

The amount an individual pays for coverage.

PRESCRIPTION DRUG COVERAGE

Health insurance that helps pay for prescription drugs and medications.

PRESCRIPTION DRUGS

Drugs and medications that by law require a prescription.

PRESENT VALUE

The price a buyer is willing to pay for one or a series of future benefits. The term is generally associated with a formal computation of the estimated worth in the future of such benefits from which a discount or compensation for waiting is deducted.

PREVENTIVE CARE

Care rendered by a physician to promote health and prevent future health problems for an individual who does not exhibit any symptoms (for example: a routine physical examination, immunizations, annual flu shot etc.).

PREVENTATIVE MAINTENANCE

The activities that are performed on a scheduled basis including adjustments, replacements, and basic cleanliness, that forestall machine breakdowns.

PREVENTIVE MEDICINE

The medical specialty that focuses on the health and well-being of individuals, communities or defined populations in order to maintain health and prevent disease, disability or a premature demise. These specialists are experts in biostatistics, epidemiology, environmental and occupational medicine, planning and evaluation of health services and the management of health care organizations

PRICE NORMALIZATION

The process of addressing differences in prices charged to different healthcare facilities for the same products by the same suppliers such that all entities pay the same price for the same product from the same supplier.

PRICE TRANSPARENCY

Most often this term refers to the ability of a consumer to discover how much a particular medical service or treatment will cost, preferably before receiving the service or treatment.

PRIMARY CARE

Routine office medical care, usually from an internist, obstetrician-gynecologist, family practitioner, or pediatrician.

PRIMARY CARE PHYSICIAN (PCP)

A doctor that provides basic care and coordinates other care through referrals to specialists as needed.

PRIMARY CARRIER

The insurance carrier which has first responsibility for payment under Coordination of Benefits.

PRIMARY PAYER

The insurer that is required to pay before a secondary insurer is asked to pay.

PRIMARY PLAN

The plan that pays first when you are covered by more than one insurance plan.

PRINCIPLE DIAGNOSIS CODE

The condition responsible for causing the admission of a patient for care.

PRIOR AUTHORIZATION

A procedure governed by a contract used to review and assess the medical necessity and appropriateness of elective hospital admissions and non-emergency care before the services are provided. Also called pre-authorization.

PRIVACY RULE

The standards for privacy regarding a patient's medical history and all related events, treatments, and data as outlined by HIPAA.

PRIVATE PRACTICE

A healthcare professional that meets all appropriate federal, state, local or regulatory body requirement's but works independently in a private setting.

PRIVILEGES

The right to provide medical or surgical care services in the hospital, within well-defined limits, according to an individual's professional license, education, training, experience and current clinical competence. Hospital privileges must be delineated individually for each practitioner by the hospital board, based on medical staff recommendations. Also called Clinical Privileges, Staff Privileges or Medical Staff Privileges

PROCEDURE

The step-by-step instructions on how to perform a specific task based on technical and theoretical knowledge.

PROCEDURE ROOM

A room for the performance of procedures that may require the use of sterile instruments or supplies but does not require an aseptic field. Local anesthesia and minimal and moderate sedation may be administered in a procedure room, but anesthetic agents used in procedure rooms must not require special ventilation or scavenging equipment. Procedure rooms are considered unrestricted areas.

PROCESS MEASURE

The series of actions or steps which lead to a certain anticipated and desired outcome.

PROCUREMENT

Acquiring by any means i.e. purchase, rental, lease etc. goods and services. Also referred to as the purchase of supplies, services and equipment from user requirement through to payment.

PROCUREMENT RECORD

Documentation of the decisions made and the approach taken in the procurement process and summarized in the Project Document and or the Purchasing department file. The documentation should indicate the adherence to the Purchasing policy and rationale for the contract award.

PRODUCT EVALUATION COMMITTEE

A multi-disciplinary committee that establishes the process by which new clinical products are introduced to the hospital and that provides a mechanism for existing products to be reviewed and analyzed. May also be called a New Technology Committee or Value Analysis Committee.

PRODUCTIVE HOURS

Total hours worked. These don't vary with patient volume. They can be either fixed or variable. An example of fixed hours are for management. An example of variable hours are for staffing.

PRODUCTIVE HOURS BY FTE

The percent of productive hours multiplied by 2080 hours.

PRODUCTIVITY

Defined as worked hours per unit of service (WHPUOS). It is calculated by taking the actual worked hours and dividing it by the volume (patients, units, visits etc.) for the same time period.

PRODUCT STANDARDIZATION

The process by which hospitals purchase a single item or product from one or two vendors.

PROFESSIONAL COMPONENT

The professional services provided to patients by hospital based physicians. This does not include any education, research or administrative functions provided by these physicians.

PROFESSIONAL FEE

The amount charged for professional services provided by individuals that are not employees of the hospital.

PROFESSIONAL MISCONDUCT

Failure of an individual to provide acceptable and ordinary skill in their profession. Also called malpractice.

PROGNOSIS

The expected outcome of a health situation.

PROGRESSIVE CARE UNIT (PCU)

The term the American Association of Critical-Care Nurses (AACN) uses to describe areas that are also referred to as Intermediate Care Units, Direct Observation Units, Step-down Units, Telemetry Units, or Transitional Care Units as well as to define a specific level of patient care. It is a unit that provides 24-hour care to adult patients diagnosed with medical cardiac conditions who require telemetry monitoring.

PROJECT DOCUMENT

Paperwork that is usually assembled by the Engineering department, which outlines the scope of work, expected deliverables, budgeted dollars and hospital signatures, for work which requires careful monitoring and inspection.

PROMPT PAYMENT DISCOUNT

A discount offered by the supplier to encourage timely payment by the hospital within the stated term identified by the supplier.

PROLONGED RELEASE MEDICINES

Medications that are slowly released into the body to reduce how fast the body absorbs the medicine. Also called extended release, modified-release, controlled-release, controlled delivery, slow release and sustained-release medicines.

PROPOSAL

A bid or written submission of a quotation by a vendor or contractor in response to a hospital's request usually in competition with other vendors or contractors. Proposals must be opened in the Purchasing department at a specific time and place.

PROPOSER

A person submitting a proposal in response to a Request for Proposal (RFP).

PROPRIETARY HOSPITAL

A hospital that is owned and operated by a corporation or a group of investors. The initial source of funding is typically through the sale of stock; profits are paid to stockholders in dividends. These hospitals are also referred to as for-profit-hospitals or investor-owned hospital. For profit hospitals pay income taxes.

PROSPECTIVE PAYMENT SYSTEM (PPS)

A payment system for reimbursing hospitals for inpatient services in which a predetermined payment rate is set for treatment of specific illnesses. The system was originally developed by the U.S. federal government for use in treatment of Medicare recipients under the Tax Equity and Fiscal Responsibility Act of 1982 (TEFRA).

PROTECTED HEALTH INFORMATION (PHI)

Usually refers to demographic information such as medical history, test and laboratory results, insurance information and other data that a healthcare professional collects to identify an individual and determine appropriate care. Also called Personal Health Information.

PROTOCOL

A precise and detailed plan, or set of steps, to be followed in a study, an investigation, or an intervention, as in the management of a specific clinical condition.

PROVIDER

A physician, hospital, pharmacy etc. that provides a medical health care service.

PROVIDER NETWORK

A group of providers (such as hospitals and physicians) who agree to a pre-negotiated price for services they provide. To get that price, a patient must be covered by a particular health plan that uses that network.

PROVIDER NUMBER

The unique identifying number assigned to the provider by the payer.

PSYCHIATRY

The medical specialty that is devoted to the science and practice of treating behavioral, emotional and mental disorders.

PSYCHOLOGY

The science of working with an individual's mental process and the effects of their behavior.

PUBLIC HOSPITALS

Facilities created and controlled by the state, county, or municipal authorities. The members of the governing board are usually elected or appointed by elected officials.

PULMONARY MEDICINE

Deals with diseases and conditions of the respiratory tract.

PURCHASE

Includes purchase, lease, renting or lease-purchase of goods and services.

PURCHASE ORDER (PO)

The signed written acceptance of the offer from the vendor. A purchase order serves as the legal and binding contract between both parties. It should include an accurate description of what is being purchased, from whom, at what price, and under what terms and conditions. A requisition becomes a purchase order (P.O.) when the order is placed.

PURCHASED SERVICE

Labor, time or effort provided by an independent contractor and involving the delivery of a specific end product.

QUALITY ADJUSTED LIFE YEARS (QALYs)

The number of years of life that are saved by medical technology or service adjusted according to the quality of those years. This is often used in cost effectiveness analysis.

QUALIFIED BIDDER (VENDOR)

Vendors that meet the business need requirements (e.g., license, delivery time frame, etc.)

QUALITY

Quality healthcare is how well a doctor, hospital, health plan, or other provider of healthcare keeps its members healthy or treats them when they are sick. Good quality healthcare means doing the right thing at the right time, in the right way, for the right person and getting the best possible clinical result.

QUALITY OF CARE

The degree to which a hospitals patient care meets accepted principles and standards of clinical practice.

QUALITY ASSESSMENT

Determination of how processes and services correspond to current standards, as well as a patient's satisfaction with the care received.

QUALITY ASSURANCE (QA) DEPARTMENT

A traditional function in hospitals and other healthcare organizations that involves the monitoring and evaluation by individuals or a department to objectively and systematically monitor and evaluate the appropriateness of patient care, and to pursue opportunities to improve patient care and resolve identified problems.

QUALITY HOSPITAL RATINGS SYSTEM

The CMS hospital rating system offers a star rating based on the 11 publicly reported measures in the Hospital Consumer Assessment of Healthcare Providers and Systems survey, which assesses patient experiences. Each year the ratings evaluate patient experiences from the prior July to the following June. The highest number of stars a hospital can receive is 5 stars and the lowest 1. Data is published for each hospital on the Hospital Compare website.

QUALITY IMPROVEMENT (QI)

A continuous process of evaluating processes and procedures in healthcare delivery and support functions and then seeking improvements in efficiency, cost-effective care and patient satisfaction.

QUALITY IMPROVEMENT ORGANIZATIONS (QIOs)

Private quality improvement contractors who work with Medicaid in all 50 states. They work with healthcare practitioners, health plans, and hospitals to analyze healthcare patterns, identify opportunities for improvement, and interpret and share information about current science and best practices.

QUALITY INDICATOR

An agreed-upon process or outcome measure that is used to determine the level of quality achieved.

QUALITY MANAGEMENT

An ongoing effort to provide services that meet or exceed customer expectations through a structured, systematic process for creating organizational participation in planning and implementing quality improvements.

QUALITY MEASURE

A quality measure, also referred to as a quality indicator or metric, is a formula that converts medical information from patient records into a rate, or percentage, that shows how well a hospital cares for its patients. Quality measures can help consumers rate the performance of hospitals, health professionals, and physicians. They include:

- Clinical process measures – what was done to get to an end result (such as giving antibiotics prior to and after certain surgical procedures).

- Clinical outcomes – what was the end result for the patient (like infection rates, mortality, and length of stay in the hospital).

- Procedure volumes – how often a procedure is done at a healthcare facility or by an individual physician.

- Structure – how care is organized.

QUALITY MONITORING

The collection and analysis of data for selected indicators that enables professionals to determine whether key standards are being achieved as planned and are having the expected effect on the target population.

QUALITY OF CARE

The degree to which healthcare services for individuals and populations increase the likelihood of desired health outcomes and are consistent with current professional knowledge.

QUANTITY

The amount or number ordered at one time.

QUANTITY DISCOUNT

The reduction in the unit price offered for large volume contracts.

QUOTATION

An offer to perform a contract to supply goods and/or services in response to a request for quotation.

RADIATION ONCOLOGY

This branch of radiology deals with the therapeutic applications of radiation for the study and management of disease, especially cancer.

RADIO FREQUENCY IDENTIFICATION (RFID)

A wireless communications technology in which specialized radio-frequency tags are placed on assets that can be read by mobile and fixed RFID readers.

RADIOLOGY DEPARTMENT

Provides a wide range of diagnostic and therapeutic procedures utilizing ionizing and non-ionizing radiation; and involving invasive, non-invasive and intra-operative techniques. Imaging services include: general radiography, fluoroscopy, ultrasound, computerized tomography (CT), nuclear medicine, mammography, bone densitometry, magnetic resonance imaging (MRI), positron emission tomography (PET), and interventional radiology/angiography.

RADIOPHARMACEUTICALS

Drugs comprised of unique medicinal formulations that contain radioactive materials called radioisotopes and are used in major clinical areas for diagnosis and/or therapeutic purposes.

RANDOMIZED CLINICAL TRIAL

A clinical trial that randomly assigns participants to two or more groups.

RAPID RESPONSE TEAM (RRT)

A group of clinicians who can rapidly bring assessment and management skills to the bedside of a patient whose condition may be deteriorating, and before he or she becomes unstable and requires emergency transfer to the intensive care unit or cardiopulmonary resuscitation.

READMISSION

A related admission to a hospital within 30 days of discharge. Readmissions are sometimes thought to indicate inferior care and poor focus on transitioning the patient upon discharge, but are often due to poor compliance with recommended care by the patient. It is regarded as a preventable event and governmental and private insurers are increasingly less willing to reimburse for such care. It is essentially a de facto continuation of that earlier hospital length of stay.

REASONABLE AND CUSTOMARY CHARGE (R & C)

Charge for health care which is consistent with the going rate or charge in a certain geographical area for identical or similar services. This is also referred to as "customary, prevailing and reasonable".

REASONABLENESS OF PRICE

A price that is compared to the quoted price of an existing purchase of a like nature.

RECOMMENDED REORDER QUANTITY

The physical amounts of an item that should be reordered to maintain an optimal on-hand supply.

RECONSTRUCTIVE SURGERY

Surgery and follow-up treatment required to correct or improve a part of the body because of birth defects, accidents, injuries or various medical conditions.

RECOVERY AUDIT CONTRACTOR (RAC)

A program established to identify overpayments and underpayments by Medicare that were paid to healthcare providers and that may not have been detected through the existing program integrity effort.

RECRUITMENT PROCESS OUTSOURCING FIRM (RPO)

A firm contracted to handle the full range of hiring duties for non-executive positions. They perform the initial contact, interviewing, reference checks and new employee orientation.

RECURRING ORDER

An order that will be placed more than once for the same good or service from the same supplier using the same order number. A standing order is a common type of recurring order.

RECYCLED MATERIAL

Goods containing recycled materials.

RED BAG WASTE

Waste that is saturated with blood or body fluids must be contained in a red bag. This is per OSHA Standards.

REFERRAL

The request for additional care, usually of a specialty nature, by a primary care physician or by a specialist needing additional medical information on behalf of the patient.

REFERRAL COORDINATOR (RC)

Operates in a team with other support staff and clinic healthcare providers. Coordinates with healthcare providers and patients to facilitate and track the referral process. In addition, initiates referrals with hospitals, specialists, and other organizations (i.e. Diagnostic Imaging, Labs, etc.) when services are authorized and educates patients and providers about insurance plans and their benefits.

REFERRAL PHYSICIAN

A physician who sends a patient to another physician for examination, surgery, or to have specific procedures performed on the patient.

REGISTERED NURSE (RN)

An individual who has studied nursing for 2, 3, or 4 years and who has passed a licensing examination.

REGISTRATION

The process of entering a new patient's personal information into the hospital computer system by creating a patient record. Patients may be registered as inpatients, outpatients, or observation patients.

REHABILITATION HOSPITAL

A specialty hospital dedicated to the rehabilitation of patients with various neurological, musculo-skeletal, orthopedic and other medical conditions following their stabilization of any acute medical issues.

REHABILITATION SERVICES

Health care services that help a person get back, improve or keep skills and functions for daily living that have been lost or impaired because they became sick, hurt or disabled. These services are often physical and occupational therapy, speech-language pathology and psychiatric rehabilitation services in a variety of inpatient and/or outpatient settings.

REIMBURSEMENT

The process by which health care providers receive payment for their services.

RELAPSE

The reappearance of or increase in symptoms within an individual that has an illness or disease after some period of improvement.

RELATIVE VALUE UNIT (RVU)

The number assigned to procedures based upon the relative amount of labor, supplies and capital needed to perform the clinical procedure. The unit value represents the cost of performing the service relative to another service.

RELEASE OF INFORMATION

A signed statement from a patient or guarantor that allows doctors and hospitals to release medical information.

REMISSION

The period of time when an individual with a long-lasting illness does not have symptoms.

REMOTE MONITORING

Monitoring of a patient located at a distance from the caregivers. Remote monitoring tools are used in hospitals, as in the case of smart beds or smart monitors or virtual ICUs. Remote monitoring tools also send alerts to a nurse's station if a patient's condition worsens.

REORDER POINT

The level at which on-hand supplies must be reordered.

REPAIR COST

The charge to restore a capital asset to its full capacity.

REPLACEMENT

The substitution of one fixed asset for another.

REPLACEMENT COST

The cost at the current list price of replacing an item.

REP-LESS MEDICAL SALES MODEL

A sales model in which the manufacturer sells their products directly to the hospital without a sales representative providing a specific set of services. This usually applies to implants where the sales representative provides no services during surgery.

REPLENISHMENT

The act of restocking depleted items or supplies.

REPORTING PERIOD

The period of time for which an operating statement is prepared.

REQUEST FOR INFORMATION (RFI)

A process from a hospital to collect written information about the capabilities of various suppliers.

REQUEST FOR PROPOSAL (RFP)

A solicitation from a hospital notifying interested parties that funds are available for selected or specified projects, research, or other undertakings.

REQUEST FOR QUOTATION (RFQ)

A formal document transmitted to a potential supplier that requests price and delivery terms on a specific item or set of items. A supplier responds to an RFQ with a quotation.

REQUEST FOR SOLICITATION (RFx)

A generic term for a competitive solicitation. The solicitation method used will be determined by the dollar amount of the requested item and the complexity of the project/product. Different types of solicitations include Request for Quote (RFQ), Request for Proposal (RFP), Invitation to Bid (ITB) and Request for Information (RFI).

REQUISITION

An internal document that a hospital department sends to the purchasing department specifying the products or services required to meet its needs or replenish inventory.

REPRODUCTIVE ENDOCRINOLOGY

The study of the maternal female hormone system, including the activities of the hypothalamus, pituitary, and ovaries from puberty through menopause as it pertains to reproduction as well as the issue of infertility.

RESECTION

Partial or complete surgical removal of a part of an organ.

RESERVE

A segregation of retained earnings that are placed in a subordinate account.

RESIDENCY

A physician that receives hospital training in a specialty, consisting of two or more years following internship.

RESIDENT (HOSPITAL)

A licensed physician that is in an advanced, supervised medical training program after graduating from medical school. Also called a House Physician.

RESIDENT (SKILLED NURSING FACILITY)

Individuals that are the recipient of care from a long term care provider i.e. a skilled nursing facility (SNF) are called residents and not patients.

RESPITE CARE

Care that is provided to a hospice patient so that the primary caregiver can get some rest.

RESOURCE-BASED RELATIVE VALUE SCALE (RBRVS)

A fee schedule for physicians used by Medicare reflecting the value of one service relative to others in terms of the resources required to perform the service. The RBRVS are calculated based on the cost of physician labor, overhead, materials and liability insurance. The resulting figures are adjusted for geographical differences and are updated annually.

RESPIRATORY CARE DEPARTMENT

The department that employs licensed respiratory therapists that are trained to assess, treat, manage, control, educate and care for patients with cardiopulmonary problems. Most departments conducts EKGs, cardiac stress tests, EEG tests, pulmonary function testing, Holter and event monitoring, provide adult and pediatric respiratory care, and testing of oxygen levels for patients admitted to the hospital and on an outpatient basis. Also called the Cardio-Pulmonary Care Department).

RESPONSIBLE PARTY

The person who pays for a patient's medical expenses, also known as the guarantor.

RESTRICTED AREA

Within a surgical suite, it is a designated space that can only be accessed through a semi-restricted area in order to protect a high level of asepsis control. Traffic in the restricted area is limited to authorized personnel and patients. All personnel are required to wear surgical attire and cover head and facial hair. Masks are required where open sterile supplies or scrubbed persons may be located.

RESTRICTED FUNDS

Includes all hospital resources that are restricted to particular purposes by donors and other external authorities. These funds are not available for the financing of general operating activities but may be used in the future when certain conditions and requirements are met. There are three types of restricted funds: specific purpose, plant replacement and expansion and endowment.

RETAINED EARNINGS (OR INCOME)

Accumulated net income, less distributions to stockholders and transfers to paid-in capital accounts. This only applies to Not-For-Profit (NFP) hospitals.

RETURN ON ASSETS

A financial measure that determines how well a hospital is performing.

RETURN ON INVESTMENT (ROI)

A measurement of the amount of positive results generated by the allocation of resources (time and money) toward a specific project or goal.

REVENUE CODE

A three-digit code used on medical bills that explains the kind of facility in which a patient received treatment.

REVENUE CYCLE MANAGEMENT (RCM)

Revenue Cycle Management encompasses the entire medical billing process that manages all claims eligibility, submission, processing and payments. In a hospital the process begins when the patient enters the facility; in a physician office it begins when the patient makes an appointment. In both situations the patient provides their name, contact information and insurance company. RCM ends when the balance on the account is zero.

REVENUE-PRODUCING COST CENTERS

Hospital departments that provide direct patient services to generate.

REVERSE AUCTION

A reverse auction is a live competitive bid which takes place at a predetermined date and time on the internet, among qualified vendors, who are pre-selected. The benefit of conducting a competitive bid by reverse auction is that bidders have a specified period of time to place a bid price against their competitors' bid price without knowing whom they are bidding against. Vendors may submit more than one price during the bidding period, with the award going to the vendor with the lowest price at the end of the bid period.

RHEAUMATOLOGY

The medical specialty devoted to diagnosis and treatment of reheumatic diseases.

RICE

An abbreviation for Rest, Ice, Compression, and Elevation.

RISK

The Strategic Procurement Department defines risks as the probability of loss (financial, reputational, physical etc.) to the hospital arising from actions of the supplier in the performance of a contract. More generally, risk is a metric that includes both the probability of an outcome occurring and the severity of the consequences if it occurs.

RISK-ADJUSTMENT

When used clinically, it is a tool to account for patient-related variation (age, sex, additional diseases) when comparing different populations of patients.

RISK MANAGEMENT DEPARTMENT

An integrated, hospital-wide program for the prevention, monitoring, and control of areas of potential liability exposure. It is the intent of a hospital risk management program to enhance the safety of patients, visitors, and employees; and minimize the financial loss to the hospital through risk detection, evaluation, and prevention.

ROBOTIC SURGERY

Minimally invasive surgery involving the aid of a robotic system.

ROGUE BUYER

Purchasing activity that is done by individuals outside of the strategic sourcing department where specific suppliers have been determined and special pricing has been negotiated.

ROUNDS

The daily visit by the attending physician and the clinical support team to all of that physician's patients on the unit. During these rounds patients are typically asked questions.

ROUTINE

Regular, usual, customary, ordinary, repetitive and every day.

RULE OUT

To "rule out" means to eliminate or exclude something from consideration. For example, a normal chest x-ray may "rule out" pneumonia. The "rule out" designation disappears once the physician makes the diagnosis.

RURAL

Hospitals not located in a Metropolitan Statistical Area.

RURAL HEALTH CLINIC

An out-patient clinic that provides primary care services and is operated in a rural setting.

SaaS (SOFTWARE-AS-A-SERVICE)

This is a licensing model that consists of a developer hosting the software and licensing it to a client using a subscription model.

SAFE PRACTICES

The standardized practices that reduce the risk of harm from the processes, practices, or systems of healthcare.

SAFETY

The avoidance of injuries to patients from the care that is intended to help them.

SAFETY CULTURE

A commitment to safety that permeates all levels of an organization from frontline personnel to top management.

SAFETY STOCK

The amount of medical and surgical supply items that are kept on-hand for emergencies.

SALARIES AND WAGES

Remuneration for services performed by employees.

SAME-DAY OR CANCELLATION RATE

This Operating Room key performance indicator measures the percentage of surgical procedures cancelled (i.e., rescheduled to another day or cancelled altogether) on the day of surgery. There is often variability in how facilities define "same-day" cancellations. Depending on the facility they could define it as follows:

- Only cancellations on the day of surgery.

- Any cancellations after 12:00 pm or 1:00 pm the day before the scheduled date of surgery.

- Only elective surgery cancellations.

- All OR cancellations.

SAME-DAY SURGERY

Surgery that doesn't require an overnight hospital stay; also called ambulatory surgery or outpatient surgery.

SAMPLE SIZE

The number of people included in a clinical study, whose characteristics are similar enough to consider them members of a larger population.

SATISFACTION MEASURES

The measures that address the extent to which patients, clinicians or others perceive their needs have been met.

SCHEDULED ADMISSION

An admission that is always scheduled in advance. It may be urgent or elective.

SECONDARY INSURANCE

Additional insurance that may pay some charges not paid by a patient's primary insurance company.

SECOND OPINION

A medical opinion provided by a second physician or medical expert, when one physician provides a diagnosis or recommends surgery to an individual.

SECURE SOCKETS LAYER (SSL)

The standard encryption system that allows for the secure transmission of data between healthcare entities and merchants i.e. suppliers, payors etc.

SECURITY DEPARTMENT

The department that provides protection and a safe environment for patients, visitors and employees.

SELF-INSURED PLAN

An organization that pays health care costs out of the organization's own pocket.

SELF-PAY

That portion of the bill that is to be paid in part of in full by a patient from his/her own resources, as it is not payable by a third party.

SEMI-RESTRICTED AREA

The peripheral support areas surrounding the restricted areas of a surgical suite. These support areas include storage areas for clean and sterile supplies, sterile processing areas, areas for storage and processing of instruments, scrub sink areas, all of the corridors to the restricted area and pump rooms.

SENIOR CARE

Care for aged individuals. It is also commonly referred to as elder care or geriatric care, and includes a wide range of care services, including help with ADLs.

SENTINEL EVENT

An unexpected occurrence involving death or serious physical or psychological injury, or the risk thereof. Serious injury specifically includes loss of limb or function. The phrase "or the risk thereof" includes any process variation for which a recurrence would carry a significant chance of a serious adverse outcome.

SEPSIS

The presence of bacteria, or other small organisms or toxins, in the bloodstream.

SHARED RISK

As hospitals shift from volume based reimbursement to value-based reimbursement it is the process by which hospitals and insurers are asking MedTech organizations, pharmaceutical companies and others to share in the payment risk for a patient encounter.

SHELF LIFE

The stated amount of time an item may be held in inventory before it becomes unusable due to technical obsolescence, because some form of deterioration has occurred or because the expiration date has been reached.

SIDE EFFECTS

Unwanted effects of a drug or treatment.

SIGMOIDOSCOPY

The examination of the rectum and sigmoid colon with an endoscope.

SINGLE-INCISION SURGERY

A surgery in which only one small (2 cm) cut is made. Example: for gall bladder removal.

SINGLE SIGN-ON (SSO)

A system in which an individual can log in once and then is able to access the system from any device in the designated service area. This eliminates the number of times an individual has to log into the system.

SINGLE SOURCE PURCHASE

A purchase of goods or services which is clearly and legitimately limited to a single source of supply. See "Sole Source".

SIX SIGMA

A methodology that provides organizations with the tools to improve the capability of their business processes and improve performance. The term derives from the statistical concept of specifying a tolerance limit on errors based on six standard deviations between the mean and the nearest specification limit.

SKILLED NURSING CARE

Services provided by licensed nurses in the patient's home or in a skilled facility.

SKILLED NURSING FACILITY (SNF)

A facility that accepts patients in need of rehabilitation and medical care that is of a lesser intensity than that received in a hospital. Patients that are discharged from a hospital oftentimes go to a SNF for further care.

SLEEP DISORDER CENTER

Provides evaluation, testing, diagnosis and treatment of sleep disorders. A typical sleep disorders center consists of several private bedrooms and a sophisticated control area that monitors brain, heart, muscle and breathing activity while patients sleep. Also called a Sleep Lab Department.

SLEEP LAB DEPARTMENT

Provides evaluation, testing, diagnosis, and treatment of sleep disorders. A typical Sleep Lab Department consists of several private bedrooms and a sophisticated control area that monitors brain, heart, muscle and breathing activity while patients sleep. Also called a Sleep Disorder Center.

SLEEP MEDICINE

The field of medicine devoted to the study and treatment of disruptions in sleeping patterns. Specialists in this field work with patients to overcome such conditions as insomnia, narcolepsy, and sleep apnea.

SLOW RELEASE MEDICINES

Medications that are slowly released into the body to reduce how fast the body absorbs the medicine. Also called extended release, modified-release, prolonged release, controlled-release, controlled delivery, and sustained-release medicines.

SOCIAL SERVICES DEPARTMENT

Provides coping assistance with the psychological, social, environmental, and financial difficulties that may arise during a patient's hospitalization. Also responsible for the coordination of discharge planning, which is a centralized program to ensure each patient has a plan for follow-up care that is required. This department is usually affiliated with the Case Management Department.

SOLE SOURCE

A purchase in which only one vendor is capable of supplying the required commodities or services. See Single Source Purchase.

SOLICITATION

The documented process of notifying prospective suppliers that the hospital wishes to receive an offer to furnish goods and/or services. The process may consist of issuing a written RFx (Request for Proposal, Request for Quotation, etc.), public advertising, and posting online notices to prospective bidders.

SPECIALIST

A physician specialist focuses on a specific area of medicine or a group of patients to diagnose, manage, prevent or treat certain types of symptoms and conditions. A non-physician specialist is a provider who has more training in a specific area of health care.

SPECIALTY DRUG

High-cost prescription medications used to treat complex, chronic conditions like cancer, rheumatoid arthritis and multiple sclerosis.

SPECIALTY HOSPITAL

Licensed hospitals that provide diagnostic and treatment services to patients with specific conditions. This includes long-term acute care, rehabilitation, children's, heart or spine. In the case of behavioral health they provide diagnosis and treatment of patients with specific illnesses.

SPECIFICATIONS

Clear and accurate description of the technical requirements of a product or service, including the procedure by which it will be determined that the requirements have been met.

SPEECH THERAPY SERVICES DEPARTMENT

Helps individuals overcome speech defects using a variety of methods.

SPEND

The total expenditure for supplies, pharmaceuticals, services, human resources and capital by the health care facility.

SPINE SURGERY

The field of medicine devoted to the diagnosis and treatment of the spine which include problems with the neck (cervical spine), mid back (thoracic spine) and low back (lumbar spine).

SPORTS MEDICINE

The field of medicine devoted to medicine concerned with the functioning of the human body during physical activity and with the prevention and treatment of athletic injuries. Doctors specializing in sports medicine help patients prevent and recover from a range of injuries - from sprained knees and back strains to broken bones and torn ligaments - suffered while engaging in sports activities.

STAFFING PLAN

The plan that ensures enough staff with the right skill set will be present on every shift to provide inpatient care.

STAFF PRIVILEGES

The right to provide medical or surgical care services in the hospital, within well-defined limits, according to an individual's professional license, education, training, experience and current clinical competence. Hospital privileges must be delineated individually for each practitioner by the hospital board, based on medical staff recommendations. Also called Privileges, Clinical Privileges or Medical Staff Privileges

STANDARDIZATION

The process of reducing the variety of products used across the hospital or healthcare entity by agreeing on the use of standard products, and contracting for those products.

STANDARD OF CARE

A legal term denoting the degree of prudence and caution required of a caregiver, used in the litigation of malpractice suits.

STANDING ORDER

An arrangement between a buyer and a supplier in which the supplier is instructed to deliver a specific good or service at a specific time interval.

STATEMENT

The printed summary of a medical bill. Also called a bill.

STATEMENT OF WORK (SOW)

A scope of work that describes the work to be performed or the services to be provided. It describes tasks, directs methodologies to be used, and sets forth the period of performance. It should contain only qualitative and quantitative design and performance requirements.

STERILE FIELD

This usually refers to the area immediately around the patient prior to a surgical procedure. Included are the surgical team and all furniture and lights in the room.

STERILIZATION

Refers to any process that effectively kills or eliminates fungi, bacteria, viruses, spores etc. or other transmissible agents usually from a surface or equipment. Sterilization can be achieved through heat, chemicals, irradiation, high pressure or filtration.

STERILE PROCESSING DEPARTMENT (SPD)

The Sterile Processing Department or as it is sometimes referred to as Central Supply, Central Services, or Sterile Supply comprises that service within the hospital in which medical and surgical supplies and equipment, both sterile and non-sterile, are cleaned, prepared, processed, stored, and issued for patient care. The primary "customer" of the SPD is the Operating Room.

STEREOTACTIC

A term that refers to precise positioning in three dimensional space.

STOCK ITEM

A supply item that is kept on-hand and in inventory.

STOCK OUT

A term that is used for a supply item that is temporarily not available. Also called an Out-of-Stock.

STRAIGHT-LINE METHOD OF DEPRECIATION

This method of allocating depreciation is a function of the passage of time and recognizes equal periodic charges over the useful life of the asset. The depreciation charge calculated by the straight-line method is not affected by asset productivity, efficiency, or degree of use. The periodic charge is computed by relating the cost of the asset, less any salvage, to the useful life of the asset.

STRATEGIC SOURCING

A component of supply chain management that continuously improves and re-evaluates the purchasing activities of the hospital or health-care entity. It comprises the following functions:

- Assessment of a company's current spend (what is bought and where?)

- Assessment of the supply market (who offers what product and services?)

- Development of a sourcing strategy (where to buy what, while minimizing risk and cost)

- Identification of potential suppliers

- Negotiation with suppliers (products, prices, availability etc.)

- Implementation of a new supply system

- Tracking the results and then beginning the assessment process again to have a never-ending continuous cycle

STUDY POPULATION

The conceptual group of people (of unknown size) represented by a specific number of participants in a clinical research study. See sample size.

SUBSPECIALTY

The specialized area within a medical or surgical specialty. For example, pulmonary medicine is a subspecialty under internal medicine.

SUPPLEMENTAL INSURANCE

A secondary policy or another insurance company that covers a patient's healthcare costs after receiving coverage from their primary insurance. Supplemental insurance policies often help patients cover expensive deductibles and copays.

SUPPLIER

A vendor of purchased goods and services. Also called a Vendor and Contractor.

SUPPLY CHAIN MANAGEMENT

A process that encompasses the planning and management of all of the activities ranging from the identification of a customer need through sourcing, product selection, negotiation with suppliers, payment, storage, distribution and redistribution to add value for patients and other stakeholders.

SUPPLY CLOSET

An area within a hospital that stores routine supplies required for patient care.

SUPPLY EXPENSE

Monies spent for supplies necessary to operate the hospital.

SUPPLIER SCORECARD

A scorecard that keeps track of all supplier performance metrics. It can be associated with various categories, depending on the supplier's role within the hospital/healthcare facility. Displayed are the suppliers name and their performance ratings. The scorecard compares a supplier's current assessment results to previous results or to the results of other suppliers. Also called a Vendor Scorecard.

SURGEON

A physician that treats injury, disease or deformities with an operation.

SURGICAL AND PROCEDURAL CARE UNITS

A unit that includes clinical procedural suites and their respective pre/post recovery rooms for patient's under-going surgery, endoscopy, interventional cardiology, interventional radiology, neuroradiology and minor procedures. The unit is specifically designed to place clinical expertise and equipment with dedicated support services in one integrated area to enhance the delivery of quality care to patients.

SURGICAL BLOCK UTILIZATION

The actual operating room time used during a case divided by the total allocated time for a surgeon.

SURGICAL INTENSIVE CARE UNIT (SICU)

An intensive care unit for post-operative surgical patients such as general surgery, neurosurgery or orthopedics. Optional specialty designations include: bariatric, cardiothoracic, gynecology, neurosurgery, orthopedics, plastic surgery, transplant or trauma surgical unit.

SURGERIES –INPATIENT

Surgical services provided to patients who stay in the hospital overnight.

SURGERIES OUT-PATIENT

Surgical services provided to patients who do not stay in the hospital overnight.

SURGERY

A wide variety of diagnostic and therapeutic surgical services are offered in most hospitals such as general surgery (hernia, hemorrhoidectomy, colon, various biopsies, gall bladder, tonsillectomy, tubal ligation, and more). Some hospitals also offer other specialty areas such as ophthalmology (cataract, eyelid), podiatry (feet) and Women's Health (gynecology, scheduled and emergent C-Sections.

SURGI-CENTER

A health care facility separated physically from a hospital that provides prescheduled outpatient surgical services.

SURGICAL DEPARTMENT

Provides diagnosis and treatment through surgery. Surgery can be performed on inpatients or outpatients.

SURGICAL SITE INFECTION

An infection that occurs following surgery in the part of the body where the surgery took place within 30 days. Sometimes these infections are minor and can involve the skin only while others are more serious and can involve tissues under the skin, organs, or implanted material.

SURGICAL SUITE

The composition of one or more operating rooms and associated areas such as the scrub room, storage areas and recovery room.

SUSTAINED RELEASE MEDICINES

Medications that are slowly released into the body to reduce how fast the body absorbs the medicine. Also called extended release, modified-release, prolonged release, controlled-release, controlled delivery, and slow release medicines.

SWING BEDS

Acute care hospital beds that can also be used for long-term care, depending on the needs of the patient and the community. Only those hospitals with fewer than 100 beds and located in a rural community, where long-term care may be inaccessible, are eligible to have swing beds.

SYSTEM ARCHITECTURE

A term that refers to the way an information system is designed and maintained.

TABULATION

A listing of all pricing, submitted by bidders, which forms a basis for comparison of proposals received and ultimate determination of the lowest qualified bidder.

TACHYCARDIA

A rapid heart rate that is usually more than 100 beats per minute.

TACHYPNEA

A faster than normal respiratory rate.

TAX IDENTIFICATION NUMBER (TIN)

The number assigned to the provider by the federal government for tax reporting purposes. Also known as the Federal Tax Number or Employer Identification Number (EIN).

TEACHING HOSPITAL

A hospital that has an accredited physician residency training program(s) and typically is affiliated with a medical school.

TELEMEDICINE

The use of medical information exchanged from one site to another using electronic communications for the health and education of patients or providers and to improve patient care. It is used to conduct medical consultations or treatments from a distance. It is a quickly growing sector and has provided access to many rural residents with limited physical access to medical services.

TELEMONITORING

The ability to monitoring patients who are not at the same location as the health care provider.

TERM DATE

The end date for an insurance policy contract, or the date after which a person no longer receives or is no longer eligible for health insurance with that company.

TERMINAL CONDITION

An incurable condition in which death is imminent, the individual is in a permanent vegetative state or a coma where death is not imminent.

TERMS AND CONDITIONS

All laws, requirements, and conditions associated with a contract or purchase order (P.O.).

TERTIARY CENTER/HOSPITAL

A large medical care institution, usually a teaching hospital that provides highly specialized medical and nursing care for medical and surgical patients.

THIRD PARTY EVALUATOR

An individual or firm that is not a principal party to an arrangement, contract, deal, lawsuit, or transaction but due to its independence and expertise, has demonstrated that it is competent in accurately assessing and offering an opinion on the fairness of the arrangement, contract, deal, lawsuit, or transaction.

THIRD PARTY INFLUENCER

Individuals or entities that can significantly shape one or more stakeholder's purchasing decision process and/or timeline but are rarely accountable for the outcome.

THIRD PARTY LOGISTICS (3PL)

Companies that specialize in performing logistics related services for its customers. This often includes warehousing, transportation and more.

THIRD PARTY PAYER

Any firm which contracts with hospitals and patients to pay for their care.

THIRTY (30) DAY MORTALITY RATE

Estimates of deaths from any cause within 30 days of a hospital admission, for patients hospitalized with one of several medical conditions or surgical procedures.

THIRTY (30) DAY RE-ADMISSION RATE

The number unplanned readmissions for any cause to any acute care hospital within 30 days of discharge from a hospitalization.

THORACIC SERVICES

Medical or surgical treatment associated with the chest.

THORACIC SURGERY

The repair of organs within the thorax or chest.

THROMBOEMBOLISM

When a blood clot breaks loose within the artery or vein and travels through the bloodstream.

THROMBOSIS

The formation of blood clot in an artery or vein.

TIME OUT

A process whereby before ever surgical procedure every member of the surgical team stops and verifies that the correct procedure is about to begin on the right site of the right patient.

TIME TO HEALTHCARE SERVICES

A measure of a healthcare organization's ability to provide incoming patients with healthcare services in a timely manner

TOTAL CHARGES

Total cost for medical services.

TOTAL COST OF OWNERSHIP

The total cost of owning a product. This includes the purchase price and the on-going operational costs.

TOTAL DISCHARGES

The total number of discharges billed by the provider for inpatient hospital services.

TOTAL MARGIN

The excess of revenue over expense and gains over losses generated from all sources.

TOTAL OPERATING EXPENSES

Total cost incurred to maintain and develop the operation of the facility during the reporting period. Includes Daily Hospital Services, Ambulatory Services, Ancillary Services, Purchased Inpatient and Outpatient Services, Research, Education, General Services, Fiscal Services, Administrative Services, Physician Professional Component Expenses, and other unassigned costs. It excludes Non-operating Expenses and Income Taxes.

TOTAL PARENTERAL NUTRITION (TPN)

A technique in which nutrients are given to a person through an intravenous infusion when they are unable to feed themselves.

TOTAL QUALITY MANAGEMENT (TQM)

Within healthcare it is an approach to the improvement of the provision of health care services based on the premise that the overwhelming majority of quality failures are the result of flaws in processes and that quality can be improved by controlling these processes.

TOXICOLOGY

A blood test to screen for the presence of commonly abused drugs such as cocaine, heroin, opium, marijuana, and amphetamines.

TRANSACTION

An event or condition, the recognition of which, gives rise to an entry in accounting records.

TRANSACTIONAL RELATIONSHIP

A non-strategic, tactical process whereby the hospital or healthcare entity buys on the basis of the lowest price, best terms and best product availability.

TRANSFER

A situation in which the patient is transferred to another acute care hospital for related care.

TRANSFUSION

The transfer of whole blood or blood products from one individual to another.

TRANSITIONAL CARE UNIT (TCU)

A unit that provides specialized care for patients who no longer require all of the resources of an acute care hospital but who are too ill to be cared for at home. Patients are typically admitted to this unit for cardiac or post-surgical recovery, pulmonary or complex medical management, oncology and pain management or skin and wound care.

TRANSPLANTATION

The transfer of living tissue or organs from one person to another.

TRANSPORTER

An individual that takes patients to their destinations via wheelchair or walking and ensures their comfort.

TRAUMA/BURN ICU

The area of the hospital which provides nursing care of the most concentrated and exhaustive nature for patients with major injuries or burns. This unit is staffed with specially trained nursing personnel and contains monitoring and specialized support equipment for patients who require intensified, comprehensive observation, and care.

TRAUMA CENTER-HOSPITAL

A facility that provides emergency and specialized intensive care to critically ill and injured patients. These hospitals are verified by the American College of Surgeons as a level I, II, or III trauma center or a level II pediatric trauma center designated by the state Department of Health.

TREATMENT AUTHORIZATION CODE

A number that indicates that the treatment provided has been authorized by the payer.

TRIAGE

A means of classification of ill or injured persons by severity of conditions. This most commonly occurs in the emergency department.

TRICARE

The health care program for members of the military, eligible dependents and military retirees. TRICARE was formerly called CHAMPUS (Civilian Health and Medical Program of the Uniformed Services).

TRIMESTER

Pregnancy is divided into three periods called trimesters. The first trimester is from the date of the last menstruation until 12 weeks. The second trimester is from week 12 to 28 and the third trimester begins at week 28 until delivery.

TRUSTEE

An individual who voluntarily serves on the Governing Board of a hospital or health system providing oversight and direction.

TUBE FEEDING

The administration of liquefied foods that are nutritionally balanced through a tube inserted into the esophagus.

TUMOR REGISTRY

Data collected on the incidence of cancers and personal characteristics, treatments and outcomes of patients diagnosed with cancer.

TURN-AROUND-TIME (TAT)

It is commonly defined as the time from when a test is ordered until the result is reported. Turnaround times can be defined differently according to the test type (stat versus routine), analyte or procedure, and institution. Within a hospital turnaround times are very important.

TWO MIDNIGHT RULE

The CMS rule that outlines the difference between a hospital inpatient and outpatient stay. It determines whether a hospital will be paid on an observation status or an inpatient status.

UB-04

The Form UB-04, also known as the CMS-1450, is the standard claim form to bill Medicare Administrative Contractors (MACs) for medical services when a paper claim is allowed.

ULTRASOUND

Ultrasound is a simple, safe, painless diagnostic procedure that bounces high-frequency sound waves off parts of the body and captures the returning "echoes" as images. There is no injection or radiation exposure associated with ultrasound. There are many different types of ultrasound exams including abdomen, carotids, venous, pelvis, thyroid, renal, scrotum, and obstetrical. Ultrasound is able to capture moving images of pelvic and abdominal structures.

UNCOMPENSATED CARE

Charity care provided by doctors and hospitals for which no reimbursement or payment is made.

UNINSURABLE

Individuals who are uninsurable and who can't get insurance coverage (or can get it only at higher rates) because of their medical history. It often refers to people who are already seriously ill when they apply for coverage.

UNITS OF SERVICE

A means to measure volume over a given period of time. Hospital departments may track different units of service to help them understand how their volume is trending. This measures the volume of work done in a department.

UNIT DOSE

A method of providing medications in individual packages for each patient by the pharmacy with each patients name, dose and schedule of delivery provided.

UNIVERSAL PRECAUTIONS

The precautions taken to prevent the transmission of blood borne diseases when first aid or healthcare is provided.

UNIVERSAL PROTOCOL

A protocol performed before every surgical procedure where the surgeon confirms the procedure with the patient and marks the body part to be operated on; and for every member of the surgical team to participate in a time out before operating to ensure that the correct procedure is about to begin on the right site of the right patient.

UNRESTRICTED FUND

Includes all hospital resources not restricted to particular purposes by donors or other external authorities. All of the hospital's resources are available for the financing of general operating activities.

URGENT CARE

Care for an illness, injury or condition serious enough that a reasonable person would seek care right away, but not so severe as to require emergency room care. Also called immediate care. The care is provided in a walk-in clinic.

URINALYSIS

A standard test upon admission to a hospital or as a component of an annual physical. It can also be ordered if an individual is experiencing abdominal pain or blood in the urine.

UROLOGY

Branch of medicine that deals with the diagnosis and treatment (both medical and surgical) of disorders of the male and female tract and male reproductive system.

UROLOGIC SERVICES

Medical or surgical treatment of the urinary tract in males and females and with the genital organs of males.

USED EQUIPMENT

Goods offered for sale which do not have a full factory warranty and which are not being rented, leased, or otherwise in the actual possession of the state agency considering the purchase at the time of the purchase transaction.

USEFUL LIFE

The actual life of a device because of obsolescence or because it is no longer adequate due to improvements in technology.

USUAL, CUSTOMARY AND REASONABLE (UCR)

Amounts charged by healthcare providers that are consistent with charges from similar providers for the same or nearly the same services in a given area.

UTILITIES

Monies spent for fuel, light, water, communications and similar products or services.

UTILIZATION

Measures of patient volume and service of time usage tracked over specific time periods.

UTILIZATION MISALIGNMENT

Any wasteful and inefficient consumption, misuse, misapplication or value mismatches that occur within a healthcare organizations supply chain.

UTILIZATION REVIEW (UR)

Evaluation of an admission, the use of ancillary services, and/or length of a hospital stay, using objective medical criteria to ensure services are medically reasonable, necessary and provided in the most appropriate setting.

VALIDITY

Whether a test or technique actually measures what it is intended to measure.

VALUE ANALYSIS

Value analysis is a process to evaluate products and services based on clinical effectiveness, patient safety, and cost.

VALUE ANALYSIS COMMITTEE (VAC)

A multi-disciplinary committee that establishes the process by which new clinical products are introduced to the hospital and that provides a mechanism for existing products to be reviewed and analyzed. May also be called a Product Evaluation Committee or New Technology Committee.

VALUE BASED PURCHASING (VBP)

Value Based Purchasing is a business practice that improves the value of health care services, where value is a function of both quality and cost. The fundamental tenet of VBP states that healthcare buyers should hold healthcare providers accountable for the quality of care provided, improved patient outcomes and complete health status and its cost. The focus of VBP is to reduce waste and inappropriate care and to reward the best performers. VBP rewards hospitals for improving the quality of care by redistributing Medicare payments to hospitals with high performance in terms of quality scores (through core measures) and experience (through HCAHPS-The Hospital Consumer Assessment of Healthcare Providers and Systems survey) at the expense of lower performing hospitals.

VARIANCE ANALYSIS

A process that determines the differences from actual and budgeted or targeted levels of performance, and identification of their causes.

VENDOR

A provider of materials, supplies, services, and/or equipment. Also called a supplier or contractor.

VENDOR CREDENTIALING

The process of establishing the qualifications of an outside supplier of goods or services to enter and conduct business within a healthcare institution. This generally includes some level of verification of certain immunizations, certifications and a training component. The representative must check in at a hospital to verify that they have been appropriately credentialed, then they are provided a badge defining which areas of the hospital they have access to. The stated goals of credentialing are to protect patient safety, keep unethical individuals out of the facility and control costs. Also called Vendor Registration.

VENDOR DEBRIEFING

The process of informing a supplier why their bid was not selected upon completion of the contract award process.

VENDOR REGISTRATION

The process of establishing the qualifications of an outside supplier of goods or services to enter and conduct business within a healthcare institution. This generally includes some level of verification of certain immunizations, certifications and a training component. The representative must check in at a hospital to verify that they have been appropriately credentialed, then they are provided a badge defining which areas of the hospital they have access to. The stated goals of credentialing are to protect patient safety, keep unethical individuals out of the facility and control costs. Also called Vendor Credentialing.

VENDOR SCORECARD

A scorecard that keeps track of all supplier performance metrics. It can be associated with various categories, depending on the supplier's role within the hospital/healthcare facility. Displayed are the suppliers name and their performance ratings. The scorecard compares a supplier's current assessment results to previous results or to the results of other suppliers. Also called a Supplier Scorecard.

VERY LOW BIRTH WEIGHT (VLBW)

A baby born weighing less than 3.3 pounds (1,500 grams) and more than 2.2 pounds (1,000 grams).

VETERANS ADMINISTRATION (VA)

A federal agency responsible for veterans including VA hospitals and veterans' benefits.

VIRTUAL ICU

A traditional ICU that has an audio-visual system installed over each ICU bed that is then continuously monitored by a physician in a remote location.

VITAL SIGNS

Measurements of body temperature, pulse rate, respiratory rate and blood pressure.

VOLUME PRICING

The reduction in the unit price offered for large volume contracts.

VOLUNTEER SERVICES

Enlists and coordinates volunteers who serve in a variety of areas including admitting, ambulatory surgery, the gift shop, etc. Also called ambassadors.

WALK-UP ORDER

Any departmental or functional area supply requests that are hand delivered to the supply location.

WATCHFUL WAITING

This is a wait and see approach used by a physician to see if treatment may be needed because the patient may get better without the treatment. The length of time for active surveillance varies according to the patient's severity of symptoms, the risks and benefits of waiting, the progression of the problem, if not treated and the individuals age and medical history. This is also called Active Surveillance.

WING

A distinct portion of the facility that is an architectural extension of the facility with a corridor connecting the two. A wing can also be a separate floor of an existing facility.

WORKER'S COMPENSATION COVERAGE

States require employers to provide coverage to compensate employees for work-related injuries or disabilities.

WORLD HEALTH ORGANIZATION (WHO)

An agency of the United Nations whose mission is to prevent the international spread of diseases, such as cholera, malaria, and poliomyelitis.

WORKING CAPITAL

The sum of an institution's short-term or current assets including cash, marketable (short-term) securities, accounts receivable, and inventories. Net working capital is defined as the excess of total current assets over total current liabilities.

WORLD CLASS

Being recognized as the best in your industry on enough competitive factors while achieving positive clinical outcomes, profit/net revenue and patient satisfaction goals.

WOUND CARE CLINIC

A facility that uses a multidisciplinary team that includes board-certified physicians and highly trained registered nurses to provide high-quality care for patients with a variety of wounds such as diabetic foot ulcers, pressure ulcers, infected wounds, chronic, non-healing wounds etc. Treatment typically includes debridement (to remove dead tissue from the wound), education on how blood sugars and nutrition can affect wound healing, management of swelling with specialized wraps and stockings to promote wound healing, treatment with advanced wound care products, total contact casts to take pressure off the foot wound, management of medications used to treat the wound and referrals for additional tests.

WRITE-OFF

This term refers to the discrepancy between a provider's fee for healthcare services and the amount that an insurance company is willing to pay for those services and that a patient is not responsible for. The write-off amount may be categorized as "not covered" amounts for billing purposes.

WRITE-OFFS

Accounts that are partially or fully uncollectable and must be written off as bad debt, charity care, etc.

X-RAY

An X-ray is a non-invasive diagnostic test that involves a low dose of radiation. An x-ray "beam" is used to produce images of various parts of the body. Because it is limited to the area of interest it is an extremely safe diagnostic tool

PART 2: HOSPITAL, PHYSICIANS & KEY HEALTHCARE PERSONNEL GLOSSARY

ACCOUNTANT

Prepares the monthly and yearly statements of income and expenses and reports for the general ledger.

ACCOUNTING MANAGER

Oversees a wide range of strategic, operational, fiscal and personnel activities within the department. Specific duties often include the management of consolidated and organizational reporting and the coordination of financial inputs and outputs within all hospital departments, service lines and business functions.

ACCOUNTS PAYABLE SPECIALIST

Responsible for a wide range of accounts payable activities. Specific duties include processing invoices into the accounts payable system, maintaining and tracking payments and auditing and reviewing reports.

ACCOUNTS PAYABLES SUPERVISOR

Directs and supervises the activities of the accounts payable department which includes maintaining records of amounts owed, verifying invoices, computing discounts, coding expense reports, preparing vouchers and issuing checks for payment.

ACCOUNTS RECEIVABLE SPECIALIST

Maximizes cash collections and the resolution of aged accounts through consistent follow up activities. Responsible for the timely billing and follow-up of assigned accounts and for ensuring all accounts are paid correctly according to insurance contract terms. Consistently identifies account deficiencies that require subsequent follow-up and ensures all deficiencies are resolved.

ACTIVITY THERAPIST/GROUP THERAPIST/RECREATIONAL THERAPIST

Individuals who provide structured group therapy, recreational/socialization activity therapy on acute psychiatric programs to support patient functioning, prepare for/prevent relapse, provide symptom management strategies, wellness support activities, therapeutic recreation, etc.

ADMINISTRATIVE ASSISTANT

Performs administrative support duties for the assigned department or service line of the hospital.

ADMINISTRATOR-SKILLED NURSING FACILITY

A licensed professional that manages the facility. They plan, organize, coordinate and direct staff to provide high quality care for their residents. They are knowledgeable of all federal, state and local laws and regulations applicable to the facility, residents, personnel and physical plant.

ADMISSIONS DIRECTOR

Oversees the inpatient and outpatient admissions department while administering policies and procedures to ensure compliance with all applicable standards. Works with medical, nursing and accounting staff to ensure proper patient placement. Designs, implements, assesses, and recommends revisions to all aspects of the admissions process.

ADMISSIONS DIRECTOR- SKILLED NURSING FACILITY

Builds and grows census and payer mix by developing relationships with a growing base of referral sources and by providing prospective patients/responsible parties with appropriate information and assistance in choosing a skilled nursing facility.

ADMISSIONS SUPERVISOR

Supervises inpatient/outpatient admissions including bed assignments. Responsible for interviewing the patient and/or relative to obtain the personal and financial data required. Confirms that all insurance benefits coverage meets standards of admission as dictated by hospital policy. Also responsible for preparation of the documentation for admission and transfer.

ADMITTING/DISCHARGE CLERK

Performs a variety of clerical tasks related to the patient admission, transfer and discharge processes. Prepares and completes the admissions and discharge paperwork ensuring proper documentation.

ADULT INPATIENT CLINICAL RESEARCH CENTER

Care location for patients who have volunteered for National Institutes of Health-funded clinical trials involving investigational drugs, devices and dietary studies.

ADVANCED PRACTICE NURSE (APN)

A generic term that describes a registered nurse (RN) who has met advanced educational and clinical practice requirements beyond the basic nursing education required of all RNs.

AGENCY NURSE

The system whereby a nurse will register or sign up with a firm and tell them what hours they are available to work. The nurses are then contacted and offered work on a shift to shift basis. Agencies can be privately owned or formed by a hospital.

ALLERGIST

An allergist-immunologist evaluates, diagnoses and treats disorders involving the immune system. Examples include asthma, anaphylaxis, rhinitis, dermatitis, eczema, and reactions to drugs, foods and insect stings. The specialist also handle immune deficiency diseases, problems related to autoimmune disease, organ transplantation, malignancies of the immune system, and management of pulmonary complications involving allergic diseases.

ALLIED HEALTH PROFESSIONAL (AHP)

A healthcare professional who is licensed, certified or registered in the state to exercise independent judgment within his/her area of professional competence and who is granted privileges to render direct or indirect medical care under the supervision of a physician member of the medical staff. Examples include nurse practitioners, certified registered nurse anesthetists, respiratory therapists, physician's assistant and others.

AMBASSADOR

Individuals that greet patients upon arrival and direct them to their destinations. They may also answer phones and answer general questions about the hospital. Also called volunteers.

AMBULATORY CARE NURSE

Provide care for patients whose stay in the hospital or surgery center is for less than 24 hours.

AMBULATORY SERVICES DIRECTOR

Oversees all ambulatory outpatient services including day surgery. Usually the director is the nurse in charge.

ANATOMIC PATHOLOGIST

A doctor that specializes in the branch of pathology which deals with the tissue diagnosis of disease. May be fellowship trained or board certified in various specialized pathologies. Specialties may include GI pathology, cytopathology, hematopathology, urological pathology etc. Using sophisticated microscopes and specialized training they examine tissues and cells taken by biopsy from patients in the clinic or during an operation. By examining these tissue sections with specialty stains, they decide whether disease is present and, if so, what effect the disease will have on the patient.

ANCILLARY SUPPORT TECHNICIAN-OPERATING ROOM

Assists physicians and other members of the surgical team by positioning patients during procedures and holding retractors during surgical procedures. Also transports patients to and from surgery, orders and stocks surgical supplies and equipment according to physician preference cards, orders and stocks sterile and non-sterile and pharmacy supplies and ensures proper inventory, pulls instruments and supplies for upcoming cases and opens sterile and intraoperative supplies for procedures under the direct supervision of Clinical Nurse Staff.

ANESTHESIA TECHNICIAN

Provides the anesthesia provider (Anesthesiologist) clinical and technical support for all surgical and pain management cases by assisting in the preparation and maintenance of the patient, monitoring devices and anesthesia delivery systems, throughout the surgical procedure.

ANESTHESIOLOGIST

Responsible for the pain management of patients during surgery, maintaining their condition during surgery and assisting in their recovery afterward. Anesthesiologists also work with patients with serious chronic pain problems and patients who have critical illnesses or injuries. They also may direct the resuscitation of patients with cardiac or respiratory emergencies.

ANESTHESIOLOGY CHIEF- DIRECTOR

Manages all of the anesthesiologists in the hospital and/or surgery center. Performs scheduling and oversees procedures.

ANESTHETIST

One who administers an anesthetic (physician, nurse, or anesthesia assistant).

ANNUAL GIFT DIRECTOR

Plans and implements the healthcare organization's campaign for annual monetary gifts from corporations and other donors. Responsible for attracting and retaining prospective donors, monitoring mailings, and analyzing past donations to ensure the annual gift giving goal is achieved.

ASSISTANT PHARMACY DIRECTOR

Assists the Pharmacy department director in their daily duties and assumes responsibility in his/her absence. Oversees pharmacists and provides pharmacy services such as compounding and dispensing medications and other pharmaceuticals.

ASTHMA COORDINATOR

Participates and coordinates in the planning development, interpretation and implementation of the Asthma program for inpatients, outpatients, and school systems. Responsible for the day-to-day operation and management of the Asthma program. Performs professional, consultative, technical, investigative, advisory and education activities for program staff, other governmental agencies, community organizations, and the general public regarding implementation of the program.

ATTENDING PHYSICIAN

A hospital physician or surgeon who has completed all required training, and is licensed to practice medicine independently without additional supervision. Attending physicians visit and treat patients regularly and often supervise students, fellows, and residents. The attending physician is ultimately accountable for the care of his/her assigned patients.

AUDIOLOGIST

Evaluates and diagnoses auditory dysfunction; evaluates hearing aid function and plans, directs, and conducts aural habilitation and rehabilitation programs.

AUXILIARY

The individual that recruits, interviews and coordinates the assignments of volunteers within the hospital. The staff work at the reception desk and in the hospital gift shop. Many also deliver flowers to patient rooms and direct /take visitors to their desired location. Also called Volunteers.

BED SCHEDULER

The primary focus of this position is the coordination of patient beds throughout the hospital and to ensure that admissions are handled promptly and that information is entered into the Health Information System in a timely and accurate fashion.

BEHAVIORAL HEALTH COUNSELOR

Provides clinical assessment and psychotherapy services for a defined patient population. Services are typically available to patients or families and may be in both inpatient and outpatient settings. Treatment is usually provided in one or more of the following areas: substance abuse, emotional and behavioral issues, eating disorders and other mental disorders.

BEHAVIORAL HEALTH NURSE

Provides age-sensitive, professional patient care on the psychiatric unit as prescribed by the physician and/or needed by the patient including treatment planning and coordination, medication monitoring, group therapy, medication education, consultation and evaluations for emergency room patients or to provide crisis management evaluations for patients on other units of the hospital. Is experienced and skilled in physical and verbal crisis intervention techniques. Also called Psychiatric Nurse.

BEREAVEMENT COUNSELOR

The individual that proves counselling to the families/caregivers of hospice patients in accordance with the interdisciplinary plan of care.

BIOMEDICAL ENGINEER

Involved in testing all medical devices used in the hospital. Advises clinicians regarding the proper and safe application of medical technology. May also perform the services of the biomedical technician.

BIOMEDICAL TECHNICIAN

Responsible for installing, repairing, calibrating, preventative maintenance, electrical safety and performance verification, bench and field service on most medical equipment at the board/module level.

BLOOD BANK DIRECTOR

Supervises all operations of the blood bank which includes the responsibility to draw, process, store, and deliver blood to hospital departments.

BLOOD BANK TECHNOLOGIST

Performs routine and specialized tests such as identifying blood types and antibodies; testing blood for viruses and investigating harmful responses of the body to blood transfusions. They also collect, separate, deliver, and store blood components; and support physicians and nurses in blood transfusion therapy.

BOARD OF TRUSTEES

The legal entity ultimately responsible for hospital policy, organization, management, and quality of care. Also called the governing board, commissioners or directors. The governing body is accountable to the owner(s) of the hospital, which may be a corporation, the community, local government or stockholders.

BUDGET BUSINESS ANALYST

Prepares operating budgets for departments or service lines based on actual performance, previous budgets, the estimated revenue and strategic plan. Reviews expenditures of requisitioning departments to ensure budget conformance. Provides variance analysis of statistics, revenues and expenses. Assists in the installation of budgetary control systems. Manages & monitors budgeting applications.

BUSINESS ANALYST

Analyzes and evaluates clinical and financial data in support of clinical service lines to reduce costs, improve quality and further the goals and objectives of hospital administration.

BUSINESS OFFICE MANAGER

Oversees the day to day activities of the hospital's business office which includes admitting and registration, patient billing and collection, third-party payer relations, and/or preparation of insurance claims.

BUSINESS OFFICE SUPERVISOR

Oversees the day to day activities of one or more functional areas within a hospital's business office such as admitting and registration, patient billing and collection, third-party payer relations, and/or preparation of insurance claims.

BUSINESS DEVELOPMENT DIRECTOR

Responsible for developing and implementing strategies for the designated service line including the clinical care, diagnostic evaluation and non-clinical functions. Provides leadership, direction and support for clinical services to ensure quality outcomes, reduce costs, and patient, physician and employee satisfaction.

BURN CARE UNIT DIRECTOR

Responsible for all aspects of care provided to patients in the burn care unit.

CAFETERIA CASHIER

Operates the cash register and serves hospital cafeteria customers.

CAFETERIA SUPERVISOR

Supervises cashiering activities within the hospital cafeteria. Maintains sales records. Prepares bank deposits. Oversees the work of other cafeteria workers for the shift and coordinates duties. Monitors the opening and closing of the cafeteria. Trains new cafeteria staff and verifies competencies.

CARDIAC CARE UNIT (CCU) NURSE

Responsible for the care and needs of patients in the CCU. This includes monitoring and reporting all pertinent information to the physician, administering prescribed medications, maintaining patient records and performing total patient care.

CARDIAC CATHETERIZATION LABORATORY MANAGER

Oversees the cardiac catheterization laboratory staff and procedures carried out at the hospital. Ensures efficient and effective lab operation.

CARDIAC CATHETERIZATION TECHNOLOGIST

Assists doctors during invasive cardiovascular procedures such as angioplasty, cardiac catheterization, and electrophysiology. Prior to surgery, the technologist is responsible for ensuring the electrocardiogram equipment is in working order, and during the procedure, the technologist will monitor the electrocardiogram readouts and keep the doctor apprised of anything considered abnormal. The technologist will also prepare the patient for the procedure by cleaning, shaving, and, in the case of cardiac catheterization for angioplasty, anesthetizing the area of insertion. Daily non-surgical duties include reading and interpreting test procedures and explaining the procedures to patients.

CARDIAC MONITOR TECHNICIAN

Performs continuous observation, interpretation, and communication of cardiac rhythms for cardiology patients under the supervision of the registered nurse.

CARDIAC SURGEON

A physician who performs procedures on the heart and great vessels. They repair or replace heart valves, widen clogged arteries, repair aortic aneurysms, and perform heart bypass surgery and heart transplants.

CARDIOLOGIST

A physician that specializes in the diagnosis and treatment of diseases of the heart. Cardiologists provide medical care to patients who have problems with their heart or circulation. Typical procedures performed include: electrocardiogram (ECG) and exercise tests to measure heart function, echocardiograms (ultrasound scan of the heart), scans of the carotid artery in the neck to determine stroke risk, 24-hour blood pressure tests, insertion of pacemakers and cardiac catheterization (coronary angiography) to see if there are any blocks in the arteries.

CARDIOLOGY DIRECTOR

Responsible for the cardiology department, which includes all the cardiologists in a hospital. Directs the staff and programs for the department to ensure the highest standards of quality and service. This position is held by a physician.

CARDIOLOGY SERVICES NURSE

Plans and implements nursing care services within cardiology services. Has a strong working knowledge of critical care and stress testing. Works collaboratively with nuclear medicine, Echo and cardiology technicians to provide ancillary procedures and care.

CARDIOLOGY SUPERVISOR

Supervises the daily operations within the cardiology department. Monitors the work of all personnel to ensure the highest quality of tests, procedures, and other aspects of patient care are performed.

CARDIOPULMONARY PERFUSIONIST

Sets up and operates the equipment designed to maintain cardiopulmonary function during surgery.

CARDIOTHORACIC SURGEON

Specializes in the diagnosis, medical management, and surgical treatment of patients with diseases affecting organs inside the thorax (the chest) which involve treatment of conditions of the heart (heart disease) and lungs (lung disease).

CARDIO-VASCULAR MATERIALS MANAGER

Monitors and supervises all technical and administrative activities of the cardiovascular supply chain, and supply chain team, including the coordinating of all purchasing activity in this area. Provides effective supply chain management with a focus on consignment management, inventory control, supply distribution, expense reduction, supply utilization, and supply standardization.

CARE COORDINATOR-COMMUNITY SETTING

Outside the hospital setting this is an evolving position with no clear accepted definition. The role is similar to a nurse navigator except that most candidates come with a social work background in lieu of nursing and there is more emphasis on keeping the patient out of the hospital by making periodic telephone calls to ensure they are receiving and taking their medications, scheduling clinical appointments for them etc. May also be called a Care Navigator.

CARE COORDINATOR-HOSPITAL SETTING

Within a hospital setting they manage the transition along the entire patient care continuum with the professional staff to ensure the care plan goals are met and patient outcomes are improved. This position is usually held by a registered nurse or advanced practice registered nurse with evidence based knowledge and training. May also be called a Care Navigator.

CARE MANAGER/UTILIZATION REVIEW CLINICIAN

Usually independently licensed social workers or advanced level registered nurses who specialize in the initial and ongoing (concurrent) authorization of patient care services by third party payers or governmental entities. May function as clinical leaders in an inpatient or outpatient environment to ensure that consumers receive covered benefits from their insurance providers and that hospital documentation complies with payer contractual requirements around length of stay, extended stay justifications, level of care determinations, etc.

CARE NAVIGATOR-COMMUNITY SETTING

Outside the hospital setting this is an evolving position with no clear accepted definition. The role is similar to a nurse navigator except that most candidates come with a social work background in lieu of nursing and there is more emphasis on keeping the patient out of the hospital by making periodic telephone calls to ensure they are receiving and taking their medications, scheduling clinical appointments for them etc. May also be called a Care Coordinator.

CARE NAVIGATOR-HOSPITAL SETTING

Within a hospital setting they manage the transition along the entire patient care continuum with the professional staff to ensure the care plan goals are met and patient outcomes are improved. This position is usually held by a registered nurse or advanced practice registered nurse with evidence based knowledge and training. May also be called a Care Coordinator.

CASE MANAGEMENT NURSE

Responsible for developing, implementing and evaluating individual patient care plans to meet an individual's health needs and promote cost-effective quality outcomes.

CASE MANAGER

Responsible for monitoring and evaluating the plan of care for individual patients, providing professional clinical skills and expertise in the assessment, planning, implementation and coordination of necessary health care services.

CENTRAL DISTRIBUTION AIDE

Provides organized and properly stocked supply carts for designated nursing areas and maintains accurate records for the movement of supplies. These supplies include but are not limited to General Medical Supplies, General Patient Need Supplies and Non-Medicated IV Solutions.

CERTIFIED NURSE AID (CNA)

Provides direct care and supervision on older adult units or med/psych units where patients may require support to complete hygiene, toileting or other activities of daily living such as bathing, transferring to bed/chair, ambulating, etc.

CERTIFIED NURSE MIDWIFE (CNM)

Assists patient with healthcare needs with their activities of daily living (ADLs) and provides bedside care-including basic nursing procedures-all under the supervision of a registered Nurse (RN) or Licensed Vocational Nurse (LVN) usually within a skilled nursing facility.

CERTIFIED NURSING ASSISTANT (CNA)

Assists patient with healthcare needs with their activities of daily living (ADLs) and provides bedside care-including basic nursing procedures-all under the supervision of a registered Nurse (RN) or Licensed Vocational Nurse (LVN) usually within a skilled nursing facility.

CERTIFIED PROSTHETIST/ORTHOTIST

A professional who creates and then fits artificial limbs, braces, or devices for patients who have deformities or injuries.

CERTIFIED OCCUPATIONAL THERAPY ASSISTANT (COTA)

Help patients develop, recover, and improve the skills needed for daily living and working. Works under the direction of occupational therapists to provide therapy to patients.

CERTIFIED THERAPEUTIC RECREATION SPECIALIST (CTRS)

Improves the well-being of individuals who have illnesses or disabilities through treatment services and recreation activities using sports, arts and crafts, dance, music, and other techniques to reduce stress, improve functioning, and build confidence in their clients.

CERTIFIED REGISTERED NURSE ANESTHETIST (CRNA)

Registered nurse who has completed additional, specialized education and training in administering anesthetics to patients before, during and after surgery or child birth under the supervision of surgeons, anesthesiologists, dentists, podiatrists or other doctors. Administers general anesthesia and provides monitored surveillance and clinical management for patients receiving local or regional anesthesia in the operative or obstetric setting. Works under the medical direction of an attending Anesthesiologist in providing anesthesia care and post-operative evaluation for patients in the Operating Room, Maternity Center, Cardiac Cath Lab, or Emergency Room setting.

CHAPLAIN

Helps families and visitors find meaning and support in their circumstances. A chaplain is usually available for pastoral visitation and/or sacramental ministry for every faith group. Chaplains are typically available 24 hours a day.

CHARGE CAPTURE ANALYST/SPECIALIST

Responsible for ensuring that all inpatient/outpatient billing charges are captured correctly. Identifies, analyzes and reconciles any and all billing errors or omissions.

CHARGE DESCRIPTION MASTER (CDM)

A list of all tests, orders or procedures performed by the hospital and billable to the patient or the patient's health insurance provider.

CHARGE NURSE

Responsible for assessing, planning, implementing, evaluating and documenting all care activities in order to deliver efficient, effective and quality patient care. The charge nurse must have the knowledge and skills needed to provide age-appropriate care, based on the assigned unit.

CHIEF ACADEMIC OFFICER

This positon is usually found in teaching hospitals. The individual focuses on promotion and direction of the research enterprise and recruitment of research intensive faculty while providing oversight of the undergraduate and graduate medical education programs.

CHIEF CLINICAL EXCELLENCE OFFICER

The person that brings patient safety, patient experience, clinical quality, performance improvement, clinical informatics, data analytics and reporting, medical management and risk management under one function.

CHIEF DATA ANALYTICS OFFICER (CDAO)

The senior hospital executive that takes responsibility for data governance, analytics initiatives and anything else related to the use of data. Because the Health Insurance Portability and Accountability Act (HIPAA), describes the ways in which patient data can be shared and who can access it the CDAO must manage governance while coordinating data processes and strategies to meet the varying needs of the institution.

CHIEF EXECUTIVE OFFICER (CEO)

The person appointed by the Governing Board or Board of Trustees to direct the overall management of the hospital. This individual is the highest ranking executive in the hospital/ health system.

CHIEF FINANCIAL OFFICER (CFO)

The person that is responsible for the overall financial administration of the organization including general accounting, data processing and financial reporting in accordance with all facility policies and procedures. The job typically includes directing the treasury, budgeting, auditing and tax accounting and real estate activities. Also called the Vice President Finance.

CHIEF INFORMATION OFFICER (CIO)

The senior information management position responsible for information strategy and overall information management. This includes programming and maintenance of all computer systems.

CHIEF INNOVATION OFFICER (CIO)

The individual that is responsible for the development, coordination & execution of an innovation and consumer strategy for the hospital/ health system. This includes looking for solutions that will help the hospital achieve more efficient and effective care delivery as well as help innovators test and develop new ideas that support strategic institutional initiatives.

CHIEF INVESTMENT OFFICER (CIO)

This is an evolving position that oversees the hospitals or healthcare systems large financial portfolio that includes endowment, pension and other funds. Responsible for the investment strategy across all of its broad, diversified assets to position the organization for profitable long-term growth and value enhancement.

CHIEF MARKETING OFFICER (CMO)

Creates a comprehensive, differentiated and effective brand strategy that provides innovative market-driven and value-added solutions. These solutions are intended to apply across the organizations target market and care continuum in order to increase revenues. They drive awareness, preference, and demand for the hospital or health system through ecommerce, customer relationship management (CRM), creative support, digital applications, market research, and marketing data analytics. Also provides pertinent market intelligence (market conditions, industry trends and customer demographics) that contributes to the organization's growth objectives and market development across the system, operating units, and affiliates.

CHIEF MEDICAL INFORMATION OFFICER (CNIO)

Responsible for facilitating the integration of clinical and technical components of information systems across all components of the hospital/system. This position also provides guidance to Information Technology staff regarding the implementation of clinical applications to ensure the needs of physicians and clinicians are met.

CHIEF MEDICAL OFFICER (CMO)

A physician member (D.O. or M.D.) of the medical staff that works in partnership to strengthen the relationship between hospital administration and the medical staff. Responsible for planning, organizing and directing the medical staff services for the entire hospital or healthcare system. Assists the medical staff in formulating standards of care and strategic direction for quality and ensures positive medical staff relations. Works to align medical staff goals with those of the hospital or healthcare system and ensures compliance with all quality, legal, and regulatory requirements. Participates in recruitment, selection, and evaluation of employed physicians, nurse anesthetists and physician assistants. Also provides resource utilization across all departments and assists with service line development along with oversight and direction of the research program and Institutional Review Board as the Institutional Officer for the IRB.

Also called Vice President Medical Affairs (VPMA).

CHIEF NURSING OFFICER (CNO)

Responsible for the operational, financial, clinical and personnel activities of all clinical services. Specific duties include directing nursing services for the facility and works collaboratively with other care providers to meet patient care needs; participating in the development/implementation of programs and services, providing leadership related to federal, state and/or accreditation regulations/ activities associated with the practice of nursing; and working with the members of the management, ancillary and care provider team to assure operational effectiveness, clinical excellence, physician, employee and staff satisfaction. Also called Vice President Patient Care Services.

CHIEF NURSING INFORMATICS OFFICER (CNIO)

Working in collaboration with the Chief Medical Information Officer (CMIO) and Chief Information Officer (CIO) The CNIO serves as the primary conduit for developing the strategic nursing informatics plan. They analyze data, create policies and procedures and serve as a champion for complex nursing projects and systems that support efficiency and effectiveness for end users. Their primary goal is advancing nursing evidence-based practice and outstanding patient care. The CNIO also provides operational oversight of EHR system design and implementation, staffing, education, change management, and performance improvement.

CHIEF OPERATIONS OFFICER (COO)

Responsible for the smooth and efficient operation of the hospital or health system including management of the profit and loss statement for the hospital's business, as well as the related resources associated with the hospital operation. Carries the responsibility for integrating the strategic plan of the organization with the operations. Provides management oversight for the development of high quality, cost effective and integrated clinical programs within the hospital. The COO acts in the absence of the Chief Executive Officer (CEO). Exercises management responsibility over the hospital ensuring efficient services that are designed to meet the needs of patients, physicians, the public and staff.

CHIEF PATIENT EXPERIENCE OFFICER (CPEO)

Develops and executes an organization wide strategy to enhance patient satisfaction and ensure there are positive interactions between healthcare consumers and the organizations staff. They champion a commitment to optimizing the patient and family experience.

CHIEF POPULATION HEALTH OFFICER (CPHO)

Designs and implements the population health strategy for a healthcare organization and guides the clinical staff through the execution of the strategy.

CHIEF RESIDENT

A resident (medical or surgical) that manages the hospital residents (physicians) assigned to them.

CHIEF STRATEGY OFFICER (CSO)

Responsible for developing, executing, communicating and then ensuring the sustainment of the hospital or health systems short-term and long-term strategic plans.

CHIEF SURGERY

The licensed physician that directs the staff and all programs within the surgical department. Works closely with all physicians and hospital personnel to ensure high quality patient outcomes and services are provided.

CHIEF TRANSFORMATION OFFICER (CTO)

The senior executive that is focused on transitioning the hospital or health system to function under risk-based payment as a population health manager. This executive typically reports to the Hospital CEO and often has a background in the operation of ambulatory care centers, health plan management, or strategic planning.

CHIEF OF STAFF

The member of a hospital medical staff who is elected, appointed or employed by the hospital to be the medical and administrative head of the medical staff.

CHILD LIFE ACTIVITY TECH

Assists patients in coping with the stress of hospitalization through assessment of the individual with normalizing activities appropriate for their developmental age.

CHILD LIFE SPECIALIST

Works with children and their families to help them cope with being in the hospital. Educated in child development. They use medical play and other activities to help the child feel more comfortable. They provide toys and games at the bedside and supervise the playroom. An individual that is certified as a Child Health Specialist has a designation of CCLS.

CIRCULATING NURSE

A circulating nurse, or circulator, is a registered nurse who monitors the surgical procedure in an operating room during surgery and assists the team in maintaining and creating a comfortable, safe environment for the patient while observing the team.

The circulator is an intermediary between the operating room staff and the rest of the hospital. They prepare the patient for the procedure and handle the preparation for the operating room before the surgery takes place to ensure the surgical room is sterile and safe for the patient. They work with scrub techs to help maintain the sterile field in the operating room and ensure it is not compromised during the procedure. They also keep the surgical area clean and organized for the scrub tech and the physician; and remove instruments and sponges as they are used during the procedure. Additional duties may include the responsibility of supervising surgical technicians, and to transport any specimens that require diagnostic testing to the laboratory.

CLAIMS EXAMINER

Responsible for supporting the case management process. Some of the responsibilities may include: communication and collaboration with injured workers (IW), employers, providers, third party administrators (TPA), attorneys, and the State Bureau of Workers' Compensation (BWC) to obtain a safe return to work (RTW) while working within BWC designated guidelines.

CLAIMS PROCESSING DIRECTOR

Directs the planning and implementation of the hospitals' reimbursement systems, their annual enrollment and eligibility, network data management, the employee benefit plans, commercial risk, capitation, Medicare Advantage Plans, special payment plans and Third Party Administrator (TPA) contracts.

CLINICAL MANAGER - PHYSICIAN OFFICE

Manages the daily activities of a medical clinic. Hires and trains support personnel, prepares the annual budget, orders clinical equipment and supplies and oversees billing practices.

CLINICAL ADMINISTRATIVE MANAGER - HOSPITAL

Responsible for managing the daily operations of a clinic section or assigned unit within a hospital. Hires and trains support personnel. Schedules employee shifts and optimizes patient flow through efficient and effective admitting and discharge functions. Also assigns patients to appropriate clinical personnel.

CLINICAL ANALYST

Responsible for evaluating data to help improve workflow and a healthcare facility's overall clinical information system. Creates the database system for a healthcare facility that provides efficiency while meeting federal regulatory standards.

CLINICAL ASSESSMENT /CRISIS SPECIALIST

Usually an independently licensed social worker or advanced level registered nurse who provides intake and crisis assessment and care management services for patients in emergency departments or acute medical floors. These staff are specifically trained to work with individuals in psychiatric or behavioral health crises, assess for and obtain authorization for inpatient care or connect individuals to community resources and organizations to resolve crises without hospitalization.

CLINICAL DOCUMENTATION SPECIALIST

Collects, analyzes and combines patient records, diagnostic results, insurance claims and other patient care related documents to enable the patient and healthcare organization to provide better healthcare for patients and to maximize reimbursement for the services that were provided.

CLINICAL EDUCATION SPECIALIST OR CLINICAL EDUCATOR

Responsible for coordinating and implementing the on-boarding and ongoing educational plan for a specific specialty service line i.e. Critical Care, Emergency Department, Medical-Surgical, Oncology, Pediatrics, Perioperative Services etc. Also coordinate in-services and education within each of the departments.

CLINICAL ETHICS SPECIALIST

Provides guidance to patients, their families, and the hospital's professional staff on ethical policy issues and concerns that arise from clinical interactions between health care professionals and patients. Provides guidance to the hospital's ethics committee for educational and case review activities and for policy formulation. Recommends policies concerning ethical issues such as "do-not-resuscitate" and "withdrawal of life-support".

CLINICAL FACILITIES PLANNER

Offers professional services related to design, construction, development, or installation of hospital buildings and facilities. Oversees construction progress and supervises construction, equipment installation and renovation projects. Works with all hospital departments to review design changes, equipment specifications or substitutions, purchasing and payment.

CLINICAL INFORMATICS MANAGER

Responsible for overseeing the daily operations of the clinical information system at a hospital. Manages and trains staff, develops and monitors budgets and ensures all systems are in compliance with state, federal and professional regulatory standards.

CLINICAL INFORMATICS SPECIALIST

Responsible for providing Informatics expertise and resources for the hospital or specialty area. This position provides on-going user training and informatics support for various project teams or committees. They support the organization's vision and direction for computer systems, process design, data management and related processes. They also serve as a liaison between the hospital or specialty area support staff and the Clinical Information System IT team to communicate user needs and facilitate system modification to meet user needs.

CLINICAL LIAISON

An individual, most often a nurse that promotes the growth of their business (long –term acute care hospital or skilled nursing facility) by calling on referral sources and explaining the services their organizations offers. They may also evaluate potential individuals for admission.

CLINICAL NURSE SPECIALIST (CNS)

A registered nurse with a graduate degree in nursing who often provides and manages the care of individuals and groups with complex health problems and provide health care services that promote, improve and manage healthcare within the nurse's specialty.

CLINICAL OUTCOMES DIRECTOR

Analyzes clinical outcomes data to develop clinical process improvement initiatives and ensure that patient care is provided in accordance with clinical guidelines and organizational standards. Defines and implements performance metrics that balance clinical and financial concerns.

CLINICAL PATHOLOGIST

A medical specialist who deals with the diagnosis of disease, based on the laboratory analysis of bodily fluids, such as blood, urine, and tissue homogenates or extracts using the tools of chemistry, microbiology, hematology and molecular pathology. The American Board of Pathology certifies clinical pathologists, and recognizes the following secondary specialties of clinical pathology: Chemical pathology, also called clinical chemistry, hematopathology, blood banking - transfusion medicine, clinical microbiology, cytogenetics and molecular genetics pathology.

CLINICAL PHARMACIST

Within the hospital clinical pharmacists are a primary source of scientific information and advice regarding the safe, appropriate, and cost-effective use of medications. They often collaborate with physicians and other healthcare professionals on the science and practice of drug administration and dosage and provide medication therapy evaluations and recommendations.

CLINICAL PSYCHOLOGIST

Individuals concerned with diagnosis and treating diseases of the brain, emotional disturbances and behavior problems. They have a doctorate in psychology and have advanced training in promoting mental health and helping people cope with problems. They use talk therapy for treatment as opposed to a psychiatry or other physician that uses medicine.

CLINICAL PSYCHOLOGY

The science of working with mental processes both normal and abnormal and their effects on human behavior, generally practiced by licensed psychologists.

CLINICAL RESEARCH DIRECTOR

Directs and oversees the clinical research function for a healthcare organization. Develops the research studies and creates standards and guidelines for all clinical research that adheres to the institutions operating procedures, clinical practice and FDA regulations.

CLINICAL RESEARCH SPECIALIST

Organizes research information for clinical projects and assists with data analysis and reporting.

CLINICAL TRANSPLANT COORDINATOR

Assumes responsibility and accountability for comprehensive care, support and education to transplant recipients, living donors and their families throughout all phases of the transplant process. Identifies and meets the physical and emotional needs of the patient, ensuring the coordination of the clinical aspects for the transplant recipient or living donor

CLINICAL UNIT SUPERVISOR

A registered nurse that oversees the day-to-day delivery of professional nursing care in a specifically assigned unit or department, ensuring that nursing care provided is consistent with established nursing standards, and provided in a safe, appropriate, and cost-effective manner.

CLINICAL SPECIALIST-RESPIRATORY CARE

The clinical specialist is usually an experienced registered respiratory therapist (RRT) who coordinates work in specialized areas, like the ICU. They are responsible for monitoring work flow, monitoring care path adherence and quality metrics, and communications with other health care professionals.

CODER

Ensures all patient treatments are coded properly for the appropriate charges for care. This individual reviews medical records and assigns the latest codes to diagnoses and procedures so healthcare facilities can bill payers and receive the correct reimbursement amount.

COLLECTIONS SPECIALIST

Responsible for ensuring the collection of past due account balances through contact of patients by phone and/or mail. Sets up alternative payment plans when necessary.

COMMUNITY LIAISON

For health systems that also offer home health care, hospice, and/or home medical equipment (HME) services, this position promotes the health system as the home care provider of choice within the communities served. The primary focus/responsibility is to increase the volume of patient referrals into their home health, hospice or HME program. They market to current and potential referral sources such as physicians, hospitals, and community groups providing support to the chronically ill and comparable referral sources and payers.

COMPENSATION ANALYST

Provides analytical and project support in the design, implementation and maintenance of compensation programs, tools and services including base pay administration, market pricing of jobs, assisting with new job evaluation requests, compensation project support and other compensation related activities in support of key Human Resource projects and initiatives.

COMPENSATION & BENEFITS MANAGER

Responsible for the development, implementation and administration of compensation and benefits for all hospital employees.

COMPLIANCE DIRECTOR

Designs and implements programs, policies, and practices to ensure that all hospital departments are in compliance with Joint Commission, HIPAA, and accreditation standards. Tracks laws and regulations that might affect the organization's policies and procedure and maintains compliance with federal, state, and local regulatory requirements. Prepares monthly compliance reports to present to senior management.

CONSULTING PHYSICIAN

A physician with an area of expertise, who may be asked by an attending physician, to help diagnose and treat a patient.

CONTINUING EDUCATION DIRECTOR

Responsible for evaluation, development, and implementation of continuing education programs for health professionals.

CONTROLLER

Responsible for all accounting, budgetary and financial planning and reporting activities within the hospital organization under the direction of the CFO. Manages the development of financial reports, including income statements and balance sheets.

CONTRACT MANAGEMENT SPECIALIST-MANAGED CARE

Administers the managed care contracts for the organization. They also participate in the development and implementation of contract management tools and processes to assist in achieving the organizations contracting objectives and strategies.

CONTRACT SPECIALIST

Responsible for analytical support and negotiation pertaining to all contracts such as contract negotiation, interpretation and guidance, ensuring compliance with all regulatory agencies.

COOK

Responsible for the preparation of hot and cold entrees for patients, cafeteria and special functions.

COST ACCOUNTANT

Responsible for procedure level costing, maintenance of the hospital's financial decision support system and maintenance of managed care contract models. Assists with accurately reconciling the cost accounting process back to the financial statements. Provides analytics as required.

COURIER/DRIVER

Drives, loads, and unloads mail, medical reports, supplies, equipment, lab specimens, pharmaceuticals, and other items within the hospital system, affiliated locations, and clinics.

CREDENTIALING SPECIALIST

Obtains all primary source information necessary for the initial and reappointment verification process for all hospital personnel requesting staff privileges. Maintains records and the integrity of highly confidential information.

CRISIS ASSESSMENT SPECIALIST

Responsible for the assessment of clients in consultation and cooperation with emergency department personnel, psychiatrists, clinicians, attending physicians and managed care representatives. Provides recommendations for patient disposition.

CRITICAL CARE SPECIALTIES

Manage patients with life-threatening conditions such as coma, trauma, heart failure, organ failure and respiratory conditions. Critical care specialists are also trained in internal medicine.

CT TECHNICIAN/TECHNOLOGIST

Responsible for a wide variety of tasks to maximize patient flow within the CT department. Specific duties may include operating the CT scanner and other support equipment, transporting patients, handling telephone calls/scheduling patients.

CYTOTECHNOLOGIST

Microscopically screens gynecologic and non-gynecologic slides containing cells from all body sites. Prepares and processes specimens and assists pathologists, radiologists and clinicians with fine needle aspirates as needed and operates, calibrates, checks and maintains instrumentation.

DATA ADMINISTRATOR

Manages and maintains a variety of data used in support of analytical and/or research projects.

DATA ANALYST

Responsible for generating and providing data and reports for the assigned department or service line.

DATA ENTRY CLERK

Performs a variety of routine data entry activities in accordance with established departmental and hospital procedures.

DECISION SUPPORT ANALYST-FINANCE

Develops, prepares, interprets and monitors financial analyses, financial projections, financial modeling, and reports used by hospital management in decision-making. Provides assistance in performing extensive data mining and abstracting of financial and clinical information from various decision support tools for capital budgeting/planning, business plan development (pro-forma, retrospective analyses), service line reporting and analyses, charge master support, revenue and reimbursement analyses, and ad hoc reporting needs of the department.

DENTIST

An individual who has received a doctor of dental medicine or doctor of dental surgery degree and is currently licensed to practice Dentistry in the state and whose practice is in the area of oral and maxillofacial surgery or an area of general Dentistry.

DEPARTMENT CHAIR

The individual or designee who is responsible for administration and oversight of his/her respective Department at the hospital.

DERMATOLOGIST

A physician who specializes in the diagnosis and treatment of benign and malignant disorders of the skin, mouth, external genitalia, hair and nails, as well as a number of sexually transmitted diseases. They provide care for normal skin to prevent skin diseases and skin cancers and diagnose and treat skin cancers, melanomas, moles, and other tumors of the skin, contact dermatitis and other allergic and non-allergic disorders.

DESKTOP ANALYST

Provides support, trouble shooting, repairs and replacement for end user computer hardware and peripherals. Also performs diagnostics, installations, removals and relocations of hardware and software and establishes screen access per user account.

DIABETES EDUCATION COORDINATOR

Coordinates the hospital's diabetes education program; assesses patients' need for diabetes care and/or education.

DIALYSIS TECHNICIAN

Sets up and operates the artificial kidney machine to provide dialysis treatment for patients with kidney disorders or failure.

DIENER-PATHOLOGIST

Interacts with clinicians, family members and funeral directors upon the death of an inpatient. The typical support provided includes: preparing the necessary paperwork, preparing the body for movement to the morgue, helping the family with any necessary arrangements, interacting with the Medical Examiner, discussing and securing permission for autopsy from the family, performing the autopsy and preparing the proper specimens for analysis. This position also has the responsibility of maintaining the gross room and frozen section area and coordinating inventory ordering, pick up and storage.

DIETARY AIDE

Responsible for collecting and checking menus, calculating patient diets and tray delivery to patients.

DIETICIAN-REGISTERED (RD)

A licensed, registered food and nutrition expert who works with patients to ensure they have the proper diet. Their duties often include counseling and instructing patients on modified diets.

DIGITAL MARKETING COORDINATOR

Responsible for planning, implementation and support of digital marketing projects such as maintaining and enhancing the website, collaborating with the Director of Marketing, Service Line Leaders, Communications Manager, copywriters and other subject matter experts both inside and outside the hospital to contribute and update content and ensure that the hospital website is up to SEO standards, optimizing web architecture, enhancing key words and editing to create copy for optimum navigation.

DIGITAL MARKETING SPECIALIST

Helps drive consumer demand and brand preference by implementing effective campaigns across the digital marketing spectrum, including conversion optimization, search engine marketing (SEM), search engine optimization (SEO), social media, email marketing and more.

DIRECTOR-AMBULATORY OPERATIONS

Plans, directs, manages and coordinates activities for a system's Family Health Center and all Department of Medicine Subspecialty Clinics. Coordinates and manages business planning, program development, marketing, and facility construction and renovation planning tied to capital projects in all practice locations. Manages daily operations, budgets and supervises staff.

DIRECTOR-ANCILLARY SERVICES

Directs and coordinates all aspects of ancillary services such as pharmacy, medical records, physical, speech and occupational therapy. Sets policies and procedures and ensures all services meet the objectives of the organization.

DIRECTOR-BEHAVIORAL HEALTH PROGRAMS

Responsible for the overall administrative and related clinical performance of the behavioral health programs at the hospital. Prepares and manages budgets, manages and supervises staff and ensures quality services are provided through daily operations. Directs performance improvement activities. Prepares and manages budgets, manages and supervises staff and ensures quality services are provided through daily operations. Directs performance improvement activities.

DIRECTOR-BIOMEDICAL ENGINEERING

Develops, directs, organizes and manages the overall operations and distribution of resources (staffing, budgets and outside vendor services) of the biomedical equipment department of the hospital. This includes review, auditing and decision support activities related to problem diagnosis, repair, preventive maintenance and quality assurance of patient care resources (staffing, budgets, and outside vendor services) of the biomedical engineering department and other assigned capital asset equipment. Prepares and manages budgets, manages and supervises staff and ensures quality services are provided through daily operations. Directs performance improvement activities.

DIRECTOR BUSINESS DEVELOPMENT

The individual responsible for all referral development activities within a long-term acute care hospital, skilled nursing facility or rehabilitation hospital. Directs the efforts of all clinical liaisons. In some organizations may also manage the inpatient admissions team.

DIRECTOR-BUSINESS OFFICE

Oversees hospital admissions, billing, collections and customer service. Assists in budget preparation, general accounting and preparation of reports. Prepares and manages budgets, manages/supervises staff and ensures quality services are provided through daily operations. Directs performance improvement activities.

DIRECTOR-CANCER CARE

Plans, directs, manages and coordinates activities for the oncology service line for infusion and supportive care services and radiation oncology services in conjunction with the Cancer Program Medical Director. This includes psycho social services, cancer screening programs, the cancer committee, tumor registry, research program, radiation therapy and medical oncology. Prepares and manages budgets, manages/supervises staff and ensures quality services are provided through daily operations. Directs performance improvement activities.

DIRECTOR-CARDIAC CATHETERIZATION LAB

Provides direction and leadership for the overall operations, quality assurance, patient satisfaction and financial management of the Cardiac Catheterization Lab, EP lab and Non-invasive Cardio Diagnostics and the Cardiac Rehab program. In collaboration with the other members of the leadership team, develops and implements strategic plans, program development and overall success of the Cardiac Cath Lab, EP lab and Non-Invasive Cardio Diagnostics program. Prepares and manages budgets, manages/supervises staff and ensures quality services are provided through daily operations. Directs performance improvement activities.

DIRECTOR-CASE MANAGEMENT

Oversees all strategic, operational, fiscal and personnel activities for the case management department. Specific duties often include the preparation and management of budgets and the supervision of staff, while ensuring quality care and service to all hospital patients. Prepares and manages budgets, manages and supervises staff and ensures quality services are provided through daily operations. Directs performance improvement activities.

DIRECTOR OF CASH MANAGEMENT

Directs the Treasury functions in establishing and maintaining consistent, accurate and timely recording and reconcilement of cash across all hospital entities. Develops and implements cash accounting policies and internal controls.

DIRECTOR, CLINICAL INFORMATION SYSTEMS

Improves the health of populations, communities, families and individuals by optimizing information management and communication. This includes the use of appropriate technology in the direct provision of patient care, establishing effective clinical information systems, planning and delivering educational experiences that support life-long learning, and creating evidence based practices.

DIRECTOR-CLINICAL LABORATORY

Responsibilities include planning, organizing and directing the overall operation of the clinical laboratory Department. Activities include the performance of chemical, microscopic and bacteriologic tests performed in the laboratory to obtain data for use in diagnosis and treatment of diseases. Additional responsibilities includes recognizing results or problems that require referral to the Pathologist, assuring competency of all personnel, formulating the budget for the department, maintaining performance improvement activities within the department and participating in CQI activities and maintaining efficient and effective departmental operations in compliance with all state, federal, and local regulatory laws, standards and protocols. Prepares and manages budgets, manages/supervises staff and ensures quality services are provided through daily operations. Directs performance improvement activities.

DIRECTOR OF COMMUNICATIONS

Provides leadership in the creation and implementation for all communication initiatives that support the hospital's patient care, education, research and service missions. Oversees and implements the external and internal communications and consults on media relations. Also designs and develops communication initiatives, materials and planning.

DIRECTOR OF COMMUNITY AFFAIRS

Coordinates all strategic community relations activities in the defined geographical area that support the marketing, communications and public affairs for the hospital's activities. Integrates public relations programs and initiatives into a cohesive effort that conveys a consistent message in support of the hospitals strategic goals and objectives.

DIRECTOR-COMPENSATION

This position is often at the corporate office of a health care system. They often manage a team of analysts and project and process managers that provides expert advice and consultation with Human Resources and services line leaders on the alignment of compensation programs with business strategies. They participate in salary surveys; analyze survey results and recommend changes to the compensation program to maintain compensation objectives and competitive position in the marketplace.

DIRECTOR-DRG CODING

Responsible for duties related to the prospective payment system (PPS), including early determination of the patient's Diagnosis Related Group (DRG); informing the attending physician of the normal length of stay, and providing additional information from the case mix index management information system. Prepares and manages budgets, manages and supervises staff and ensures quality services are provided through daily operations. Directs performance improvement activities.

DIRECTOR OF ELECTRONIC HEALTH RECORD (EHR) SYSTEM

Responsible for implementing the electronic health record system (EHR) for the hospital. Accountable for all aspects of planning, staffing, training, and budget monitoring for the initiative. Acts as the primary liaison between key legacy system staff, operational leadership and the end-user community.

DIRECTOR-EMERGENCY SERVICES

Directs patient care duties of professional and non-professional personnel and programs of the emergency services department to promote the effective and efficient utilization of personnel. Provides triage and treatment to pediatric, adult and geriatric patients seeking emergency care. Develops and introduces approved standards and guidelines for emergency service programs. Ensures quality care for patients. Prepares and manages budgets, manages/supervises staff and ensures quality services are provided through daily operations. Directs performance improvement activities.

DIRECTOR-ENVIRONMENTAL SERVICES/HOUSEKEEPING

Manages the daily operations of the housekeeping department to ensure all areas of the facility are kept in a clean and orderly condition. Supervises staff, procedures, scheduling, and purchasing of housekeeping and janitorial services and supplies. Ensures that all infection control standards are met. Also responsible for the implementation of an integrated waste management program including infectious and bio hazardous waste disposal, recycling and waste prevention programs, linen distribution and collection. Typically is responsible for all areas within the hospital especially patient rooms, clinics and physician offices assigned to them. Prepares and manages budgets, manages/supervises staff and ensures quality services are provided through daily operations. Directs performance improvement activities.

DIRECTOR-FACILITIES MANAGEMENT

Responsible for the continuous and uninterrupted operation and maintenance of the hospital and all owned medical office buildings, waste treatment, clinical air and vacuum, fire alarm and fire-fighting systems, electrical distribution and emergency provisions. This includes maintenance of all buildings and equipment in a state of proper repair, preventive maintenance on all equipment and of parking lots and grounds. Provides long range planning and programming for future development and expansion of services, including financial, environmental and safety implications. Responsible for the department meeting accreditation standards, complying with hospital policy and procedures, managing supplies and equipment. Prepares and manages budgets, manages/supervises staff and ensures quality services are provided through daily operations. Directs performance improvement activities.

DIRECTOR OF FINANCE

Directs and coordinates the preparation of the operational budgets for the hospital and owned entities; directs monitoring of fiscal operations for compliance with the approved budget; and implements the hospitals policies and guidelines as they relate to budget and payroll.

DIRECTOR-FINANCIAL OPERATIONS & REPORTING

Responsible for leadership and oversight of financial operations and reporting for a health system. This includes integrity and compliance (which includes the completeness and accuracy) of all internal and external financial reporting on a monthly, quarterly and annual basis. Also ensures all financial statements are in accordance with Generally Accepted Accounting Principles (GAAP) and for the compliance and coordination of all audit requirements, plus tax and other regulatory filings including form 990s and the Cost Report.

DIRECTOR-FOOD SERVICES

Oversees the food service department and plans, directs and coordinates the therapeutic diets and food service for patients and hospital employees. Is also responsible for the handling, storage and preparation of food and supplies, maintenance of equipment, records and sanitation in accordance with health requirements and standards. Prepares and manages budgets, manages/supervises staff and ensures quality services are provided through daily operations. Directs performance improvement activities.

DIRECTOR-FUND RAISING

Responsible for all fund raising, donations and endowments for the hospital.

DIRECTOR-HEALTH INFORMATION MANAGEMENT (HIM)

Responsible for the management of all operations of the department and its computer systems. Functions as an organizational resource person on health information management issues including release of information, confidentiality, information security, information storage and retrieval, and record retention as well as authorship and authentication of health record documentation, standardization of medical vocabularies, and use of classification systems. Prepares and manages budgets, manages and supervises staff and ensures quality services are provided through daily operations. Directs performance improvement activities. Also called Director of Medical Records.

DIRECTOR-HUMAN RESOURCES

Responsible for partnering with the hospitals leadership team in overseeing all aspects of human resources functions including recruitment, staff relations, orientation, organizational and leadership development, compensation and benefits, as well as managing workers' compensation and compliance with OSHA regulations. In addition, the HR Director develops and recommends human resources practices and procedures that assist in the growth and talent management of the hospital and is responsible for ensuring compliance with federal, state and local laws and regulations. Prepares and manages budgets, manages/supervises staff and ensures quality services are provided through daily operations. Directs performance improvement activities.

DIRECTOR-INFECTION CONTROL

Manages the hospital's program of infection control including sanitizing, cleaning, disinfecting, decontaminating, and sterilizing medical products and devices that are essential to safe patient care and staff welfare. Coordinates all aspects of the facilities infection control program. Is directly involved with programs that prevent and control healthcare-acquired infections. Serves as an infection control consultant for facility staff. Interacts with physicians and outside agencies as well as all departments within the facility. Prepares and manages budgets, manages and supervises staff and ensures quality services are provided through daily operations. Directs performance improvement activities.

DIRECTOR-INFORMATION TECHNOLOGY (IT) ADMINISTRATION

Coordinates IT staffing and recruiting; identifies process improvement opportunities; prepares the department's annual operating and capital budgets; monitors and reports on performance against the budget; oversees the purchasing and invoice processing and payables functions for IT and functions as part of the management team for the IT department.

DIRECTOR-MANAGED CARE CONTRACTING

Responsible for a defined market's managed care contracting. Typical activities include the identification of opportunities to improve financial and market share performance, analysis, maintenance, negotiation and renegotiation and management of all agreements with current and prospective purchasers and providers of healthcare services. Also coordinates the communication of managed care contracts and their requirements with all hospital departments. Prepares and manages budgets, manages and supervises staff and ensures quality services are provided through daily operations.

DIRECTOR-MARKETING

Develops and directs marketing strategies to increase utilization and revenue of the hospital/system, services and service lines based on organizational business goals and objectives through marketing and public relations. These can include advertising, educational outreach, internal communications, etc. Also responsible for directing and implementing the hospital/system brand strategy. Prepares and manages budgets, manages and supervises staff and ensures quality services are provided through daily operations.

DIRECTOR-MATERNITY SERVICES

Responsible for the daily operation of the maternity unit, which includes labor, delivery, recovery, postpartum, and the baby nursery. Is often responsible for community outreach educational programs and women's health initiatives. Prepares and manages budgets, manages/ supervises staff and ensures quality services are provided through daily operations. Directs performance improvement activities.

DIRECTOR-MEDICAL STAFF CREDENTIALING

Responsible for managing the verification process for all hospital personnel requesting staff privileges. Develops and implements policies and protocols related to physician, nurse and other employee verifications to ensure the hospital and staff are in accordance with organizational and industry standards. Maintains records and the integrity of highly confidential information.

DIRECTOR-NEUROLOGY

A licensed physician that directs the staff and programs of the neurology department. Directs the staff and programs for the department to ensure the highest standards of quality and service.

DIRECTOR-NURSING

Directs and administers strategic, operational, fiscal and personnel activities for the hospital nursing department in accordance with established regulatory agencies. Prepares and manages budgets, manages and supervises staff and ensures quality services are provided through daily operations. Manages clinical operations and development with measurable improvements in clinical outcomes and customer patient satisfaction. Prepares and manages budgets, manages/supervises staff and ensures quality services are provided through daily operations. Directs performance improvement activities.

DIRECTOR-OBSTETRICS & GYNECOLOGY

A licensed physician that directs the staff and programs of the obstetrics and gynecology (OB/GYN) department. Directs the staff and programs for the department to ensure the highest standards of quality and service.

DIRECTOR-OCCUPATIONAL THERAPY

Oversees all aspects of occupational therapy which includes organizing and conducting medically prescribed therapy treatment to individuals with developmental, physical, cognitive and/or emotional impairments, disabilities and/or handicaps, with the goal of helping the patient attain a maximum level of independence and performance. Prepares and manages budgets, manages and supervises staff and ensures quality services are provided through daily operations. Directs performance improvement activities.

DIRECTOR-OUT-PATIENT SURGERY (SAME-DAY SURGERY)

Responsible for the day-to-day operation of the out-patient surgery center. Creates, directs, and implements their policies and procedures and ensures a high level of quality care and services for patients by coordinating staff and physicians. Directs performance improvement activities.

DIRECTOR-OUTPATIENT SERVICES

Supervises and coordinates all of the activities of the personnel that manage the out-patient departments and clinics. Prepares and manages budgets, manages and supervises staff and ensures quality services are provided through daily operations. Responsible and accountable for developing, implementing, and integrating performance improvement plans. Assures implementation and maintenance of departmental and hospital policies, procedures and standards of care. Assures all state and federal laws are in compliance in areas of responsibility. Assures all Joint Commission standards are followed in areas of responsibility.

DIRECTOR-PERIOPERATIVE SERVICES

Plans, organizes, supervises and coordinates the Perioperative Service department that includes the Operating Room, PACU, Pre-Admissions, Day Surgery and Sterile Processing. Prepares and manages budgets, manages/supervises staff and ensures quality services are provided through daily operations. Directs performance improvement activities.

DIRECTOR-PHARMACY OPERATIONS

Oversees the operation and administrative direction of Pharmacy Services. Specific duties include the implementation and administration of unit policies and procedures, preparation of financial and operational analyses and reports, and the oversight of current systems in order to identify opportunities for improved efficiency. The Director is also responsible for the education of healthcare professionals and patients with regard to medication use, along with compounding and dispensing prescribed medications for patient care. Prepares and manages budgets, manages and supervises staff and ensures quality services are provided through daily operations. Directs performance improvement activities.

DIRECTOR-PHYSICAL THERAPY

Manages all aspects of the hospital's physical therapy program including rehabilitation, patient services, etc. Prepares and manages budgets, manages/supervises staff and ensures quality services are provided through daily operations. Directs performance improvement activities.

DIRECTOR-PRODUCT DEVELOPMENT

Responsible for managing the development, enhancement, and roll-out of strategic product lines as well as project schedules and deliverables. Brands and successfully implements new products such as an Accountable Care Organization.

DIRECTOR-PUBLIC RELATIONS

Organizes and directs public relations activities to ensure the hospital has a favorable image with the community and hospital staff.

DIRECTOR-QUALITY IMPROVEMENT

Directs and administers strategic, operational, fiscal and personnel activities for the Quality Department. Prepares and manages budgets, manages and supervises staff and ensures quality services are provided through daily operations. Directs performance improvement activities.

DIRECTOR-RADIOLOGY/DIAGNOSTIC IMAGING

Oversees all operations in the Radiology department such as X-rays, EKGs, ultrasound, and radiology procedures. Hires and trains radiologic technologists, orders the necessary equipment and manages the budget of the department. Ensures their institution complies with all state and federal regulations. Prepares and manages budgets, manages/supervises staff and ensures quality services are provided through daily operations

DIRECTOR-RECRUITMENT

Responsible for the hospital's recruitment strategy and personnel including clinical and non-clinical recruitment personnel and support staff. Coordinates relationships with external staffing agencies, external recruitment firms, and collaborates to identify and develop strategies for hard-to-fill positions or special case recruitment scenarios and sourcing strategies.

DIRECTOR-REIMBURSEMENT

Responsible for the implementation of various strategic value added reimbursement initiatives for the hospital/health care system that includes evaluation, planning, coordination and follow through to completion of such initiatives as: Wage index reviews, Medicare Bad Debt optimization strategies, Medicaid Eligible Days reviews, various cost based optimization strategies, and any reimbursement methodology related to Medicare and Medicaid that have reimbursement implications.

DIRECTOR-RENAL DIALYSIS

Responsible for the day to day operation of the renal dialysis department. Manages the treatment of hemodialysis, peritoneal dialysis and other services. Prepares and manages budgets, manages/ supervises staff and ensures quality services are provided through daily operations

DIRECTOR-REVENUE CYCLE MANAGEMENT

Directs and oversees the overall policies, objectives, and initiatives of the hospital's and owned medical groups revenue cycle activities (i.e. Patient Access, Billing and Collections). Reviews, designs and implements processes surrounding pricing, billing, third party payer relationships, collections and other financial analyses to ensure that the clinical revenue cycle is effective and properly utilized. Maintains revenue cycle KPI's within established industry and/or organizational standards and motivates, facilitates, mentors and coaches everyone to deliver high quality, cost effective services. Prepares and manages budgets, manages/supervises staff and ensures quality services are provided through daily operations

DIRECTOR-RESPIRATORY CARE (TECHNICAL DIRECTOR)

Plans, directs, organizes, leads, and coordinates the day-to-day operation of the Respiratory Care Department. Develops and implements policies and procedures which are consistent with Joint Commission, OSHA, CLIA, state and local requirements. Often oversees pulmonary function lab and provides in-services for staff to include safety, infection control, and quality assurance. Works with hospital administration to develop long range planning, budgeting and staffing. Contributes and participates in all committees, as well as the management of employees and payroll for the Respiratory Care Department. Prepares and manages budgets, manages/supervises staff and ensures quality services are provided through daily operations

DIRECTOR-RISK MANAGEMENT, PATIENT SAFETY & REGULATORY COMPLIANCE

Responsible for the evaluation, oversight and management of patient safety, risk management, patient relations and regulatory standards. Supports the hospital mission and values through activities to protect all assets and resources of the hospital. Oversees patient grievances in an appropriate and timely manner and protects the rights of the patient and the clinical and medical staff of the organization. Also acts as a resource for the hospital regarding issues of patient safety and rights, regulatory standards and creates benchmarks for patient safety and identifies strategic initiatives to support the hospital's goals. Prepares and manages budgets, manages/supervises staff and ensures quality services are provided through daily operations

DIRECTOR-SOCIAL SERVICES

Provides assistance with the psychological, social, environmental, and financial difficulties that may arise during a patient's hospitalization. Also assesses patient and family psycho-social and discharge planning issues relevant to medical treatment. Provides crisis intervention, emotional support, resource information, discharge planning, and legal reporting. Arranges case conferences and facilitates bio-ethical consultations. Prepares and manages budgets, manages/supervises staff and ensures quality services are provided through daily operations

DIRECTOR-STERILE PROCESSING SERVICES

Responsible for the department that provides sterile medical and surgical instruments and supplies. Plans, directs and coordinates all the activities involved in the acquisition, decontamination, storage, assembly, cleaning and sterilization of medical, surgical and related supplies, materials and equipment utilized in the care and treatment of hospital patients and the operation of the Hospital Sterile Processing Department. Interfaces regularly with Operating Room staff, advising physicians, nurses and other personnel regarding products, supplies, equipment, services, instrumentation, and other issues necessary to perform designated patient care medical and surgical procedures. Prepares and manages budgets, manages/supervises staff and ensures quality services are provided through daily operations

DIRECTOR-STRATEGIC BUSINESS DEVELOPMENT

Responsible for the identification, evaluation, development and support of the implementation of new businesses that will serve to enhance the overall effectiveness and fiscal viability of the hospital/system. Provides direction and guidance to hospital/system management and service line leaders in developing sound strategies for the hospital and service lines.

DIRECTOR-SUPPLY CHAIN SPECIAL PROCEDURES

Responsible for the oversight and direction for the functions and operations of, inventory control, supply distribution, supply ordering, and financial accounting of supplies for all Special Procedure areas across all entities of the hospital including all offsite clinics and procedure centers. Participates in negotiations for supplies and equipment with objective of obtaining the best cost benefit ratio and determines the most appropriate distribution or inventory control process and systems. This includes consignment inventory.

DIRECTOR-SURGICAL SERVICES-OPERATING ROOM

The nursing position that is responsible for leading and managing all the surgical services areas including Preadmission Testing, Ambulatory Surgery, Surgery, Surgery Scheduling, Recovery Room, Anesthesia, Gastroenterology, Sterile Processing and Central Supply. Prepares and manages budgets, manages/supervises staff and ensures quality services are provided through daily operations

DIRECTOR-VALUE ANALYSIS

Responsible for leading a system wide value analysis process with the goal of providing high quality, efficient and cost effective services. Establishes and adheres to a streamlined method for standardizing and monitoring product and service selection, utilization that facilitates supply expense management while continuously improving quality, safety and satisfaction. Ensures that the teams achieve annual target savings goals while representing supply chain management and system-wide needs.

DIRECTOR-VOLUNTEERS

Organizes and directs a program for training and utilization of volunteer workers who contribute their services to supplement the work of the regular hospital staff.

DISCHARGE PLANNING DIRECTOR

Sets up the discharge schedule for patients, schedules home visits if needed, and gives patients prescriptions. Manages a staff of discharge planners.

DISCHARGE COORDINATOR-PLANNER

A healthcare professional that facilitates a patient's movement from one healthcare setting to another, or to home. It is a multidisciplinary process that involves physicians, nurses, social workers, and possibly other health professionals as required.

DISHWASHER

Performs dish washing; tray/cart transportation, trash removal and kitchen cleaning.

DOSIMETRIST

Designs and customizes treatment plans under the direction of the radiation oncologist. Also calculates radiation treatment dose and enters data into the record and verify system.

DRG CODING MANAGER

Ensures that all medical records are coded properly according to government regulations and the patient's diagnosis and treatment to allow for proper payment. Monitors data quality to ensure proper reimbursement is received.

ECHO ULTRASOUND TECHNICIAN

Performs standard and complex echocardiography procedures including stress echo, transesophageal echocardiograms, and vascular testing. Also provides technical expertise to maintain, enhance, and advance departmental standards. Assists in quality control and quality assurance.

EDUCATION COORDINATOR

Responsible for orientation of new hires, annual staff competencies, monitoring achievement of required CEUs for licensure and development of new policies and procedures. This position often exists in Nursing and Respiratory Care.

EEG TECHNICIAN

Operates and maintains electroencephalographic (EEG) machines recording brain waves on a graph to be used by physicians in diagnosing brain disorders.

EKG TECHNICIAN

Operates the computerized electrocardiogram (EKG) analysis system to record, store, retrieve, analyze, and produce a final report for all EKG's done at the hospital.

ELECTRICIAN

Constructs, installs, modifies, maintains and repairs electrical appliances, systems, facilities, and related electronic controls and devices within the hospital and associated facilities in accordance with blueprints, specifications, established practices and pertinent state and local electrical codes.

ELECTROPHYSIOLOGIST

A cardiologist who specializes in the electrical system of the heart. They perform diagnostic electrophysiology testing to find and assess arrhythmias, radiofrequency catheter ablation, and implantation of devices such as pacemakers and defibrillators.

EMERGENCY DEPARTMENT NURSE

Provides nursing care for assigned emergency room patients. These nurses quickly assess the needs of each patient, prioritize care based on its critical nature, and work to stabilize the patient, treat the problem and discharge the patient after the emergency is over or make arrangements for a longer hospital stay.

EMERGENCY DEPARTMENT PHYSICIAN

A physician who specializes in the area of emergency medicine. The emergency physician's role is to assess; treat, admit, or discharge any patient that seeks medical attention. They take a full patient history, perform a physical exam, and order and obtain the tests necessary to ascertain the cause of the patient's complaint. Upon making a diagnosis, the physician must either treat the patient or refer him/her for the appropriate follow up care. A trained emergency physician is able to handle traumas and acute and non-acute problems.

EMERGENCY DEPARTMENT REGISTRATION CLERK

Arranges for the efficient and orderly registration of patients, ensures that accurate patient information is collected and patients are aware of hospital payment policies and procedures.

EMERGENCY MEDICAL TECHNICIAN (EMT)-PARAMEDIC

Provides pre-hospital evaluation, treatment and transportation of sick and/or injured victims of all age groups. They typically operate in non-emergent, emergent and /or transfer situations at a Basic to Intermediate Life Support level, when required, until arrival at a hospital.

EMPLOYEE SERVICES MANAGER

Responsible for managing all of the employee health service functions of the hospital. Often responsible for administering employee physicals and may provide consultation regarding workers' compensation, infection control or other employee health related issues.

ENDOCRINOLOGIST

A physician that provides specialty care for patients with diabetes, thyroid disease, cholesterol disorders, pituitary disease, reproductive disorders, adrenal tumors, hyperparathyroidism, obesity and metabolic bone disorders, including osteoporosis.

ENDOSCOPY TECHNICIAL

Assists the nurse in caring for patients in the endoscopy setting, assisting the physician during endoscopic procedures and for cleaning/maintaining equipment used in the endoscopy procedure.

ENTEROSTOMAL THERAPY NURSE

Provides acute and rehabilitative care for patients from birth through all stages of life, with select disorders of the gastro-intestinal, genito-urinary and integumentary systems. Also serves as a clinician, educator, consultant and researcher; while collaborating with physicians, health care providers and ancillary departments in organizing care; and incorporating the patient's family or significant others within the care environment.

ENVIRONMENTAL SERVICES ASSOCIATE-HOUSEKEEPER

Responsible for a wide range of cleaning and service tasks within the facility. Performs a variety of heavy cleaning tasks to maintain patient rooms, offices, hallways and other assigned areas of the facility. Performs cleaning and floor refinishing functions following established protocols to achieve quality standards and facility objectives. Operates a variety of floor care equipment and other necessary tools, products and supplies. Gathers and disposes of trash and waste materials. Also called a Janitor or Environmental Services Technician.

ENVIRONMENTAL SERVICES SUPERVISOR

Supervises the operational, technical, and personnel activities within the Environmental Services Department. Manages the department's use of labor, supplies, vendors and inventory levels within budget guidelines while assuring optimal service to all clinical and non-clinical departments within the hospital.

ENVIRONMENTAL SERVICES ASSOCIATE

Performs a wide range of housekeeping tasks. Specific duties may include mopping, finishing and buffing floors; vacuuming and shampooing carpets; cleaning and restocking patient/resident rooms, nursing stations, lounges, restrooms, offices and clinic areas.

EXECUTIVE DIRECTOR-NURSING HOME ADMINISTRATOR

Directs the day-to-day functions of the skilled nursing facility in accordance with current federal, state, and local standards, guidelines, and regulations that govern nursing facilities to ensure that the highest degree of quality care can be provided to all residents. Also called a Skilled Nursing Facilitator Administrator. Prepares and manages budgets, manages/supervises staff and ensures quality services are provided through daily operations

EXERCISE PHYSIOLOGIST

Coordinates, plans and directs preventative and rehabilitative health care for patients in the Cardiovascular and Pulmonary Rehabilitation Programs by assisting the patients in achieving their optimal functional capacity through exercise, education, and risk factor modification.

FAMILY PRACTICE/PRACTITIONER

A family practitioner is a licensed physician who has completed a family practice residency and is board certified or eligible. Their scope of practice includes children and adults of all ages.

FAMILY REPRESENTATIVE

An advocate responsible for serving as a liaison between patient and family members, hospital staff, and medical staff. The Family Representative acts as a neutral party and assists families in accessing the health care system and outside community resources.

FELLOW

A physician who has completed training as an intern and resident and has chosen to continue training toward a specialty. A fellow has been granted a stipend and position allowing him or her to do further research in that chosen specialty. (Specialties include cardiology, endocrinology, infectious disease, neurology, etc.)

FLIGHT PARAMEDIC-MEDEVAC

The Flight Paramedic is an EMT Paramedic who performs medevac transport missions and who performs other activities, following the order of a physician and who conforms to approved medical protocols, while supporting and assisting the Flight nurse.

FINANCIAL ACCOUNTANT

Performs professional accounting using generally accepted accounting principles (GAAP). Reviews and analyzes various sources of information for month end journal entry preparation and posting. Prepares audit schedules and work papers for interim and year end audits. Prepares internal and/or external surveys and reports necessary to meet the requirements of federal, state, and local regulatory agencies. Prepares budget files and assists in the analysis and review of departmental budget variances.

FINANCIAL ANALYST

Responsible for financial reporting and analysis which involves: management reporting, financial modeling, and financial impact analysis. The work relates to the reporting and analysis of billing and revenue generated through accounts billed. May be asked to perform special projects such as product line profitability reporting, physician based reporting, length of stay and utilization expense reduction projects, business planning data requests, system enhancements etc.

FINANCIAL COUNSELOR

Responsible for a wide range of administrative tasks for the inpatient and/or outpatient settings. Specific duties include assessing and reviewing accounts to ensure appropriate reimbursement; providing a resource to various parties for resolution of patient financial responsibility; and recommending/approving community service.

FLOOR FINISHER

Responsible for daily floor care and finishing.

FOOD SERVICES SUPERVISOR

Supervises the food services staff and often participates in food preparation activities.

FOOD SERVICES WORKER

Prepares and delivers meal trays to patients, and then cleans up afterward. May also assist in food preparation.

GASTROENTEROLOGIST

A physician that specializes in treating conditions of the digestive system, including the stomach, bowels, liver and gallbladder. They provide diagnostic and therapeutic assistance, and also consult with surgeons when surgery is necessary.

GASTROENTEROLOGY NURSE

Provides care to patients with known or suspected gastrointestinal (GI) problems who are undergoing diagnostic or therapeutic treatment and/or procedures. They practice in hospitals, physician offices, inpatient and outpatient endoscopy departments and ambulatory endoscopy centers.

GENERAL ACCOUNTING MANAGER

Responsible for the general accounting functions of the hospital and in the preparation of reports and statistics that show earnings, profits, surpluses or losses, cash balances and other financial results.

GENERAL SURGEON

Although surgery has become increasingly specialized over the years, general surgeons still perform many procedures. They include surgeries involving abdominal organs, (such as gall bladder, stomach and bowels), some cancer and some vascular system procedures. Many times general surgeons are able to perform surgeries using laparoscopy, a minimally invasive procedure that makes treatment and recovery easier for the patient.

GENETIC COUNSELOR

Provides genetic counseling to individuals and families who are at risk for hereditary disorders. May recommend genetic testing after a discussion of the risk, benefit, and cost. Also provides crisis intervention regarding unexpected genetic conditions.

GERIATRICIAN

A physician with specialized training in the diagnosis, treatment and prevention of disorders (disease or disability) in older people. They are primary care physicians who are specially trained in the aging process. in older people.

GERIATRIC NURSE

Geriatric Nurses provide care for elderly patients in hospitals, skilled nursing facilities and their homes.

GERIATRIC PSYCHIATRY

A physician that provides care and treatment for the psychological needs of the elderly population.

GERONTOLOGIST

An individual that studies old age and aging and its effect on individuals and cultures. They are not physicians.

GIFT SHOP ATTENDANT

Assists the gift shop manager with the operations of the hospital gift shop.

GIFT SHOP MANAGER

Manages the operations of the hospital gift shop.

GOVERNING BODY-BOARD

The legal entity ultimately responsible for hospital policy, organization, management, and quality of care. Also called the governing board, board of trustees, commissioners or directors. The governing body is accountable to the owner(s) of the hospital, which may be a corporation, the community, local government or stockholders.

GRADUATE MEDICAL EDUCATION DIRECTOR

Directs the daily activities of the hospital's graduate medical education (GME) programs. Ensures compliance with the American College of Graduate Medical Education (ACGME) and ensures that medical and surgical resident work meets all their requirements. Continuously monitors medical and surgical resident assignments and scheduling. Generates reports to support the programs' ongoing accreditation.

GROUNDS KEEPER

Responsible for all grounds maintenance of the hospital and its facilities including lawn care, snow removal etc.

GYNECOLOGIST

A physician that specializes in treating diseases of female reproductive organs and providing care to keep women healthy.

HAND SURGEON

Surgeons that deal with problems of the hand, wrist, and forearm with and without surgery. Hand surgeons are typically orthopedic, plastic, or general surgeons who have an additional year of training in surgery of the hand. They treat a variety of conditions from carpel tunnel syndrome to the reattachment of fingers.

HEALTH CARE RECRUITER

Responsible for the recruitment and on-boarding of exempt and non-exempt employees, including nursing, allied health, administrative, management and support staff.

HEALTH COACH

The individual that motivates and educates patients to engage in a sustainable behavioral change so that they can achieve their health related goals.

HEALTH EDUCATION NURSE

A nurse that teaches people how to lead healthier lives. They work in a variety of settings such as hospitals, nonprofit organizations and private businesses. Health Educators may work one-on-one with patients and their families. They may teach people about wellness through classes, workshops and conferences.

HEALTH INFORMATION MANAGEMENT ANALYST/SPECIALIST

Responsible for the accurate and legal maintenance of both inpatient and outpatient medical records through the effective and efficient management of patient demographics, encounters and clinical information. This includes, but may not be limited to, managing the electronic master patient index (EMPI), investigating, validating, and resolving patient accounts/encounters as it relates to the electronic health record.

HEALTH INFORMATION DATA INTEGRITY SPECIALIST

Supports the correction of duplicate medical record numbers, cross domain merges and contact mover errors. Maintains the integrity of the electronic medical record.

HEALTH INFORMATION MANAGEMENT DIRECTOR

Combines business and computer expertise with health information management to link health care clinicians with information technology. Serves as the conduit between patients' health information and health insurers, state and federal government, and other regulating agencies.

HEALTH INFORMATION MANAGEMENT SYSTEM TECHNICIAN/SPECIALIST

Responsible for the maintenance and preservation of confidential electronic health records. The position performs a variety of functions i.e. record completion, transcription coordination, document imaging, release of information, and/or providing services and information to physicians and staff. This position may also analyze the electronic medical records for quantitative and qualitative completion based on the hospital medical staff rules and regulations, hospital policy, and State, Federal and other regulatory agency requirements.

HEART TRANSPLANT SURGEON

Examines, diagnoses, and surgically treats patients with end-stage heart disease by surgically replacing a diseased or damaged heart with a healthy heart.

HEMATOLOGIST

Physicians that treat diseases of the blood, spleen and lymph nodes. They manage conditions such as anemia, sickle cell disease, hemophilia, leukemia and lymphoma. They also perform biopsies and transfusions.

HEMODIALYSIS CLINICAL NURSE

Delivers nursing care to patients in the dialysis unit including observation and treatment of patients and documentation of treatment and progress.

HIPAA COMPLIANCE SPECIALIST

Performs various activities to ensure compliance with federal and state laws and hospital policies related to the privacy, security, and confidentiality of healthcare information consistent with regulatory, contractual, and ethical requirements. Conducts HIPAA-related audits including but not limited to those that are routine, directed, and complaint driven and ensures they are handled appropriately, and timely. Also works closely with Information Systems personnel to analyze applications, hardware, software, IS infrastructure, storage, transmission, connectivity, etc. for HIPAA compliance.

HISTOLOGIST

The scientist that specializes in the structure, composition, and function of cells and tissues.

HISTOTECHNOLOGIST/HISTOTECHNICIAN

Histology Techs are allied health professionals employed in the clinical laboratory with advanced training that provides them with the ability to perform technical procedures to provide results to the pathologists for rendering diagnosis. These procedures are performed according to established and approved policies that are in compliance with the College of American Pathologists standards. They prepare slides from tissue sections for microscopic examination and diagnosis by the pathologist and operate computerized laboratory equipment to fix, dehydrate, and infiltrate with wax, tissue specimens to be preserved for study by the Pathologist.

HIV/AIDS Nurse

Nurses that provide healthcare for patients who are HIV or AIDS positive.

HIV Specialist

A physician that specializes in the diagnosis and treatment of HIV patients and HIV associated conditions.

Home Health Agency Nurse

A registered nurse who visits patients in the home and provides hands-on care while educating the patient and family on the treatment and the prevention of future episodes.

Home Health Aide

For healthcare organizations that provide home health care this position provides personal care and related non-professional household services necessary to meet the hygiene, activities of daily living, and comfort needs of the homebound patient.

Home Health-Clinical Director

Ensures quality and safe delivery of home health services by coordinating services that reflect the facility's philosophy and standards of care. Also plans, develops, implements and evaluates services, programs and activities. Not all hospitals have a home health program.

Home Health Internal Transition Coordinator

Oversees patient transition from on-site care to in-home health care.

Hospital Greeter

Welcomes patients, family and visitors as they enter the main hospital and helps them find a particular service or unit. Also called an Information Desk Assistant or Volunteer.

Hospital Interpreter

Over 24 million Americans do not speak good enough English to communicate effectively with their healthcare provider. Interpreters provide an accurate translation to the language of the listener. They foster accurate and complete communication between the patient and the healthcare worker. Hospital interpreters can assist during an examination, procedure, admission, consultation, or other provider-patient encounters. Federal law requires hospitals that receive Medicare, Medicaid and other government funds to provide interpretation services free of charge.

HOSPITALIST

A hospital based physician. Hospitalists assume the care of hospitalized patients in the place of the patient's primary care physician. Their responsibilities include patient care, research, and leadership related to hospital care.

HOUSEKEEPER

Responsible for a wide range of cleaning/service tasks within the facility. Performs a variety of heavy cleaning tasks to maintain patient rooms, offices, hallways and other assigned areas of the hospital. May perform cleaning and floor refinishing functions following established protocols to achieve quality standards and facility objectives. May operate a variety of floor care equipment and other necessary tools, products and supplies. Gathers and disposes of trash and waste materials. Also called a Janitor or Environmental Services Associate.

HOUSE PHYSICIAN

A medical trainee (intern or resident) who has completed medical school, but is still undergoing the required training to be licensed to practice medicine independently.

HOUSE SUPERVISOR

A registered nurse is responsible for a wide range of administrative and patient flow activities. Specific duties may include pre-admission clinical arrival information, along with coordination of patient transfers, resource utilization and management, and operations for all clinical and non-clinical departments during an assigned shift. Responds to facility emergency situations and initiates the disaster notification process if required.

HUMAN RESOURCES (HR) MANAGER

Serves as consultant for rewards and recognition, performance management, recruitment/ retention, policy development and interpretation, dispute resolution/mediation communication and payroll transactions to assigned areas of responsibility.

HUMAN RESOURCES SPECIALIST

Advises and assists management and employees on employee issues and concerns by communicating, interpreting and recommending appropriate use of human resource policies and procedures, services and programs.

HYPERBARIC TECHNICIAN

Performs hyperbaric oxygen (oxygen delivered at pressures above sea level atmospheric pressure) therapy on approved patients under the direction of a physician. Operates and monitors the hyperbaric chamber.

IMMUNOLOGIST

Scientists or clinicians who study an organism's defense (immune) system, in both health and disease.

INFECTION CONTROL NURSE/MANAGER/PRACTITIONER

Provides patient safety that is focused on hospital-wide infection surveillance, control and prevention. Acts as a resource and consultant to all clinical services, support services, management services and medical staff regarding organizational infection prevention and control. Coordinates comprehensive system-wide infection prevention and control program and activities.

INFECTIOUS DISEASE SPECIALIST

Physician that specializes in the diagnosis and treatment of infections due to viral, bacterial, fungal or parasitic causes; for example, Lyme disease, hepatitis and malaria.

INFORMATICS NURSE

Nursing Informatics is a broad field which combines in-depth (specialty) nursing knowledge with the use of computers. They help determine what IT applications will increase efficiency. They train the clinical staff on new systems and technology. They also facilitate communication between IT, vendors and the hospital staff regarding clinical IT applications.

INFORMATION DESK ASSISTANT

Welcomes patients and family/visitors as they enter the main hospital and help them find a particular service or unit. Also called a Hospital Greeter or Volunteer.

INFORMATION TECHNOLOGY PROJECT MANAGER

Provides project management and/or coordination for hospital / department projects. Responsibilities include project and task planning with subject matter experts and application area project managers, effort and resource estimating, time tracking, status reporting and deliverable management.

IN-SERVICE EDUCATION DIRECTOR

Organizes classes and training sessions for internal staff members of the hospital.

INSURANCE VERIFICATION SPECIALIST

Responsible for the pre-verification of insurance for patients being admitted into the hospital for care. Ensures insurance coverage and resolves any issues with coverage and escalates complicated issues to a supervisor or manager. Interviews patients and completes all paperwork necessary to ensure the admitting process is efficient and all hospital and regulatory policies are in compliance.

INTENSIVE CARE UNIT /CRITICAL CARE UNIT DIRECTOR

Oversees all aspects of the ICU/CCU, including budgeting and employees.

INTENSIVE CARE UNIT (ICU) NURSE

Responsible for the care and needs of assigned patients in the intensive care unit.

INTENSIVIST

A physician that specializes in the care of critically ill patients, usually in an intensive care unit.

INTERNAL MEDICINE CHIEF

Oversees the internal medicine department. This branch of medicine deals with diagnosis and medical (non-surgical) therapy of disorders and diseases of the internal structures of the body.

INTERN

A physician who is in the first year of medicine after graduating medical school. An intern is sometimes called a "first year resident." They are not yet licensed to practice medicine independently. Interns and residents gain practical experience with patient care in a hospital setting, while under the direct supervision of more senior, board-certified physicians. They are now more commonly called Post Graduate Year, or PGY I, II, III, IV or V or a House Physician.

INTERNIST

Another name for a physician that specializes in internal medicine. Physicians that provide patients with long-term comprehensive care. Internists are trained to handle simple and complex illnesses, for patients of all ages. They are considered primary care providers (PCPs), with training in emergency internal medicine and critical care.

INTRAVENOUS INFUSION CENTER

Adult outpatient center that provides a variety of tests and / or IV medications for the diagnosis or treatment of chronic medical conditions such as Oncology, Pulmonary, Gastroenterology, Endocrinology, Hematology, Nephrology, Transplant, Cardiology, Hepatology, Ophthalmology, Genetics, Infectious Disease, Dermatology, Rheumatology, Neurology or General Medicine services. Patients are released to home or to a long term care facility at the end of their procedure.

INTERVENTIONAL CARDIOLOGIST

Performs minimally invasive procedures using small catheters and incisions instead of surgery. These procedures include balloon angioplasty to open blocked arteries, balloon valvuloplasty to widen a stiff or narrowed heart valve, implantation of coronary stents to hold open previously blocked arteries and cardiac catheterization.

INVENTORY CONTROL TECHNICIAN

Maintains inventory records and associated accounts to ensure accurate records of stock on hand, and proper payment to vendors for materials received and accuracy of assigned accounts.

JANITOR

Responsible for a wide range of cleaning/service tasks within the facility. Performs a variety of heavy cleaning tasks to maintain patient rooms, offices, hallways and other assigned areas of the hospital. Performs cleaning and floor refinishing functions following established protocols to achieve quality standards and facility objectives. May operate a variety of floor care equipment and other necessary tools, products and supplies. Gathers and disposes of trash and waste materials. Also called a Housekeeper or Environmental Services Associate.

LABOR & DELIVERY NURSE

Nurses that provide care for women during labor and childbirth, monitoring the baby and mother, coaching mothers and assisting doctors.

LABORATORY MANAGER

Oversees and coordinates the daily operation and activities for the laboratory. Plans and implements policies, procedures and services for a laboratory unit and/or the work shift.

LABORATORY MEDICAL TECHNOLOGIST

Responsible for routine and specialized laboratory testing such as hematology, special chemistry, blood bank, microbiology, serology, and urinalysis and quality control. Often rotates in various sections of the clinical laboratory as assigned.

LABORATORY TECHNICIAN

Receives and processes specimens, distributes specimens to technical areas, assists technical staff in retrieving stored specimens and often dispatches phlebotomists to patient care areas to draw specimens. Complies with Occupational Safety and Health Association, hospital and laboratory safety management plan, departmental policies and procedures, and safe work practices.

LACTATION CONSULTANT

A coach, consultant, teacher, and lactation expert that works with the Birthing Center, Newborn and Intensive Care nurseries, Pediatrics, OB, Family Practice, and nursing care teams to develop feeding plans for a range of infants from the normal newborn to the complex neonate.

LAUNDRY ASSISTANT

Receives clean linen and stocks exchange carts and par level storage areas. Uses forms and portable data collection devices to monitor and control linen usage. Prepares soiled linen for internal cleaning or retrieval by the contract linen company.

LAUNDRY MANAGER-SUPERVISOR

Directs the activities of service personnel, revises schedules and coordinate all aspects of linen services within the healthcare facility. Supervises the receiving, washing, ironing, packaging and delivery of the laundry within the hospital.

MAGNETIC RESONANCE IMAGE (MRI) TECHNOLOGIST

Operates the magnetic resonance scanner to obtain images for use by physicians in the diagnosis and treatment of pathologies.

MAINTENANCE ELECTRICIAN

Operates and maintains technically sophisticated electrical equipment. Trouble shoots and performs preventative maintenance on electrical and electronic (including analog and digital) systems.

MAINTENANCE MECHANIC

Operates and maintains technically sophisticated mechanical equipment. Troubleshoots and performs preventative maintenance on pneumatic, and mechanical equipment.

MAINTENANCE TECHNICIAN/WORKER

Responsible for providing basic building maintenance, preventative and corrective work required for the hospital. Building maintenance activities typically include general fire alarm systems, hospital beds, TVs, plumbing, medical gas outlets, nurse call systems, pneumatic tube system, elevators, furniture, fixtures and equipment. Works with and assists other tradesmen in completing required tasks.

MAMMOGRAPHY TECHNICIAN/TECHNOLOGIST

Provides mammographic imaging. Explains the mammography procedure and evaluates the image for technical quality.

MARKETING & COMMUNICATIONS MANAGER

Develops, coordinates, implements and supervises the hospital's marketing and community relations programs to ensure the hospital's community presence and achievement of strategic goals. Often assists in the fundraising efforts of the hospital.

MARKETING MANAGER

Leads a team that builds strategic marketing, advertising, and media campaigns. Responsible for market intelligence through identification and analysis of internal and external data relevant to the market as well as an assessment of the "competitive" environment. Leads primary and secondary market research initiatives and manages vendor or agency relationships. Measures and reports outcomes; responsible for assigned marketing budgets.

MATERNAL & FETAL MEDICINE SPECIALIST

A physician that specializes in high-risk pregnancies to protect the mother and baby. They are an obstetrician/gynecologist who has completed 4 years of Obstetrics & Gynecology training followed by 2-3 years of additional education and clinical experience in maternal-fetal medicine. Also called a Perinatologist.

MATERIALS MANAGEMENT ASSOCIATE

Coordinates supply needs to ensure adequate supply levels are available to meet the needs of all hospital departments. Also provides administrative support for Receiving, Distribution, Central Service, Linen, Par Stock, Copy Center, and Mailroom.

MATERIALS MANAGEMENT BUYER

Purchases supplies, capital equipment and purchased services to ensure an uninterrupted flow of goods at prices consistent with hospital standards for quantity, quality, safety and efficiency. Ensures that all efforts are exhausted to obtain quality product or service, on-time and at the best price. Also called a Purchasing Buyer or Strategic Procurement Buyer.

MEDICAL ASSISTANT

An allied health practitioner that assists physicians in their office. Depending upon the practice they can take patient histories and vital signs, records the information and assists in the patient's examination or treatment. Also prepares the treatment rooms for patients.

MEDICAL BILLER

Compiles the amounts owed a hospital or healthcare provider. Maintains all patient payment records.

MEDICAL DIRECTOR-LABORATORY

A pathologist, either Clinical or Anatomic that has an administrative focus for one department. May also have clinical or anatomic pathology responsibilities.

MEDICAL INTERPRETER

Provides interpretation for Limited English Proficient (LEP) patients and their families. This position acts as a conduit of information between healthcare providers and patients and families.

MEDICAL LIBRARIAN

Acquires, organizes, maintains and provides the reference collection for the medical professionals and medical staff. Catalogs, indexes, issues books/materials, and keeps records of items on loan. Also selects books and publications for purchase and subscribes to pertinent medical journals.

MEDICAL OFFICE MANAGER

Responsible for overseeing the day-to-day operations of a physician practice at either one or multiple sites including employee scheduling and development, Information Systems, physician scheduling, maintenance of medical records and files, quality management, office billing and collections, purchasing supplies and managing expenses. Also called a Physician Office Manager.

MEDICAL ONCOLOGIST

A physician that specializes in the diagnosis and treatment of cancers, as well as benign tumors. They select and administer chemotherapies, and work closely with surgeons and other specialists in caring for patients.

MEDICAL RADIATION PHYSICIST

This individual typically works in a hospital's radiology department or cancer center. Within a radiology department they are in charge of the use of diagnostic equipment such as X-ray machines. They ensure the device is correctly calibrated to give a safe and effective dose and they are in charge of measuring how much radiation the devices in the radiology department expend, and for ensuring that staff and visitors are protected from any unnecessary or excessive exposure. Within the hospital's oncology department they are responsible for the safety and correct use of radiation treatments for cancer patients. They work with the other members of the oncology department to design treatment plans that will avoid exposing patients to excessively high or frequent doses of radiation. They are also responsible for maintaining radiation safety standards to protect the people who work in the oncology department, and for checking the equipment continuously to make sure the correct dose of radiation is being used.

MEDICAL RECORDS TRANSCRIPTIONIST

Individuals who listen to recordings by physicians and other healthcare professionals that dictate a variety of medical reports and who then type them into the medical record or other documents as required.

MEDICAL RECORDS TRANSCRIPTIONIST SUPERVISOR

Assigns, schedules and oversees the work of the transcription area of the Medical Records department. May occasionally work as a Transcriptionist depending on workload.

MEDICAL RESIDENT

An individual that has received a medical degree and who practices medicine under the supervision of fully licensed physician usually in a hospital or clinic.

MEDICAL SECRETARY/MEDICAL ADMINISTRATIVE ASSISTANT

Provides secretarial support to clinical staff usually within a clinic or physician office. Answers telephones, screens callers, relays messages, and greets visitors. Types routine correspondence and reports from dictation or handwritten copy. Often obtains pre-certifications required by health care insurers or managed care providers. Informs patients of the costs for care being provided.

MEDICAL SCRIBE

Charts the interactions between physicians and clinical personnel and their patients in real-time and then organizes the healthcare data in a way that maximizes the delivery of clinical care in an efficient and productive manner.

MEDICAL STAFF

The hospital's organized component of physicians, podiatrists and dentists that are approved by the Governing Body or Board of Trustees and granted specific clinical privileges for the purpose of providing adequate medical, podiatric and dental care for the patients of the hospital.

MEDICAL STAFF CHIEF

The physician who oversees the entire medical staff and is responsible for medico-administrative affairs. Also called the Medical Director or Vice President of Medical Affairs.

MEDICAL STAFF COORDINATOR

Provides highly knowledgeable and skilled administrative support to medical staff departments and committees by acting as a liaison between medical staff members, quality specialists, administrative and other hospital personnel and ensuring all medical staff issues are acted upon appropriately by chairmen of the various medical staff committees.

MEDICAL STAFF CREDENTIALING COORDINATOR

Collects and analyzes verification data and documents for initial appointments and reappointments to the Medical Staff according to hospital and outside regulatory standards as a function of the hospitals risk management function. Coordinates and conducts orientation and criminal background checks for new physicians.

MEDICAL STUDENTS

Individuals who are in training to become physicians. The first two years are called preclinical training. During years three and four they work under close supervision and do not make independent decisions about diagnosis or treatments.

MEDICAL TECHNOLOGIST-CHEMISTRY TECHNOLOGIST

Performs clinical laboratory procedures, quality control/assurance and instrument maintenance and troubleshooting under the supervision of a lab supervisor and/or manager. The medical technologist is responsible for reporting test results to patient care units so that laboratory services consistently provide high quality patient care.

MENTAL HEALTH TECH/MILIEU THERAPIST

Usually bachelor's level unlicensed staff who provide direct supervision, para-professional counseling, patient education and safety on acute psychiatric units. These staff usually carry out nurse or physician directed intervention, supervision of high risk patients and are specially trained to manage and intervene in behavioral health emergencies. Techs may vary in training and certification from those directly licensed by the state to those with on-the-job training in behavioral health and experience. In most environments, techs also provide didactic groups, such as community meetings or recreational and socialization activities not considered psychotherapy.

MICROBIOLOGIST

Performs and demonstrates proficiency in areas including aerobic and anaerobic bacteriology, mycobacteriology, mycology, virology, fluorescent microscopy and parasitology.

MILITARY NURSE

Military Nurses work in family practice at a local military base or in a military hospital.

NAVIGATOR

The individual that is focused on specific populations and diagnoses. They facilitate patient and family health and treatment activities in collaboration with a healthcare facility and payers.

NEONATOLOGIST

A physician that specializes in the care of newborn infants.

NEONATAL CARE DIRECTOR

Oversees care of newborn babies. This position is held by a physician i.e. a neonatologist.

NEONATOLOGY/PERINATOLOGY ICU NURSE

Provides nursing care to neonatal patients within the neonatal intensive care unit.

NEPHROLOGIST

A physician that specializes in the diagnosis and treatment of kidney-conditions and (renal) disease. They routinely consult with surgeons about kidney transplantation.

NETWORK ENGINEER

Responsible for maintaining, deploying and monitoring the hospital or healthcare system data network infrastructure. Specific duties includes updating network documentation, routine maintenance, conducting utilization studies and the establishment of fault notification procedures.

NEUROLOGIST

A physician that specializes in the diagnosis and treatment of kidney conditions and (renal) disease. They routinely consult with surgeons about kidney transplantation.

NEUROLOGY SURGEON

Examines, diagnoses, and surgically treats disorders of the brain, spine, spinal cord, and nerves. Usually operates on the brain in order to relieve pressure from an intracranial hemorrhage, to remove a tumor, treat a wound, or relieve pain. They operate on the spine to free ensnared nerves, correct a deformity, or restore spine stability.

NEUROSCIENCE NURSE

Provides care for patients with diseases of the nervous system.

NEUROSURGEON

A physician that performs surgeries related to the spine and brain. The most common surgery is disc repair, to remedy back problems. Brain surgeries include removal of blood clots and tumors.

NEUROSURGERY CHIEF

Oversees the neurosurgery department. Responsible for surgery on the brain and spinal cord. This positon is held by a neuro-surgeon.

NOCTURNIST

A hospitalist that works the night shift. It is a physician that is board certified in internal medicine.

Non-Physician Practitioner (NPP)

Health care providers such as nurse practitioners, clinical nurse specialists, and physician assistants who practice either in collaboration with or under the supervision of a physician and state law.

Nuclear Medicine Manager

Responsible for managing the Nuclear Medicine staff and unit activities to ensure the production of quality studies, quality patient care, and optimal outcomes.Works with the use of radioactive materials in diagnosing and treating disease. Ensures proper usage, maintenance and updates of all equipment. May perform the duties of a technologist as needed.

Nuclear Medical Technologist

Operates the radioscopic equipment to produce scanograms and measures concentrations of radio-isotopes in specific body areas and body products for use by the physician in treating illness. Also prepares the isotopes for administration to the patient.

Nuclear Pharmacist

A registered pharmacist with 4,000 hours of training/experience in a nuclear pharmacy practice and who has achieved a passing score on the Nuclear Pharmacy Specialty Certification Examination. These individuals have advanced knowledge and expertise for the procurement, compounding, quality control testing, dispensing, distribution and monitoring of radiopharmaceuticals used with PET scans and other diagnostic procedures. They also prepare medications, troubleshoot problems with scans, and consult on health and safety issues concerning radiopharmaceuticals, as well as the use of non-radioactive drugs and patient care.

Nuclear pharmacists are employed in an institutional nuclear pharmacy connected to a major medical center/hospital where the preparations are made on-site or in a commercial centralized nuclear pharmacy where radiopharmaceuticals are prepared and then delivered to the hospital and/or clinic.

Nurse Anesthetist- Certified Registered (CRNA)

Registered nurse who has completed additional, specialized education and training in administering anesthetics to patients before, during and after surgery or child birth under the supervision of surgeons, anesthesiologists, dentists, podiatrists or other doctors. Administers general anesthesia and provides monitored surveillance and clinical management for patients receiving local or regional anesthesia in the operative or obstetric setting. Works under the medical direction of an attending Anesthesiologist in providing anesthesia care and post-operative evaluation for patients in the Operating Room, Maternity Center, Cardiac Cath Lab, or Emergency Room setting.

Nurse Clinician

A registered nurse that has received advanced training in a nursing specialty and who is allowed to practice, teach, consult, supervises or coordinate nursing services within that training specialty.

Nurse, Licensed Practical (LPN)

An individual qualified by an approved program in practical or vocational nursing and licensed by the state who, under the direction of a head nurse or nursing team leader, performs a variety of assigned nursing activities.

Nurse Manager-Behavioral Health Care

Provides clinical management and operational direction for the daily operation, activities and personnel for the Behavioral Health/ Substance Abuse units. Their duties may include scheduling and staffing, documentation, performance improvement and budgetary compliance along with staff development, physician relationships, quality initiatives, program development, and system-wide success.

Nurse Manager-Cancer Center

Provides clinical management and operational direction for the daily operation, activities and personnel for the Radiation Therapy and Medical Oncology center and staff. Their duties may include scheduling and staffing, documentation, performance improvement and budgetary compliance along with staff development, physician relationships, quality initiatives, program development, and system-wide success.

Nurse Manager-Cath Lab

Provides clinical management and operational direction for the daily operation, activities and personnel for the Cath Lab. Their duties may include scheduling and staffing, documentation, performance improvement and budgetary compliance along with staff development, physician relationships, quality initiatives, program development, and system-wide success.

Nurse Manager–ICU/Critical Care Unit

Provides clinical management and operational direction for the daily operation, activities and personnel for the ICU/Critical Care Unit. Their duties may include scheduling and staffing, documentation, performance improvement and budgetary compliance along with staff development, physician relationships, quality initiatives, program development, and system-wide success.

Nurse Manager-Maternity

Provides clinical management and operational direction for the daily operation, activities and personnel for the Maternity Unit. Their duties may include scheduling and staffing, documentation, performance improvement and budgetary compliance along with staff development, physician relationships, quality initiatives, program development, and system-wide success.

Nurse Manager-Medical/Surgical Unit

Provides clinical management and operational direction for the daily operation, activities and personnel for the Medical/Surgical Unit. Their duties may include scheduling and staffing, documentation, performance improvement and budgetary compliance along with staff development, physician relationships, quality initiatives, program development, and system-wide success.

Nurse Manager–NICU

Provides clinical management and operational direction for the daily operation, activities and personnel for the Neonatal Intensive Care Unit (NICU). Their duties may include scheduling and staffing, documentation, performance improvement and budgetary compliance along with staff development, physician relationships, quality initiatives, program development, and system-wide success.

NURSE MANAGER-PERIOPERATIVE SERVICES

Provides clinical management and operational direction for the daily operation, activities and personnel for Perioperative Services. Their duties may include scheduling and staffing, documentation, performance improvement and budgetary compliance along with staff development, physician relationships, quality initiatives, program development, and system-wide success.

NURSE MANAGER–PICU

Provides clinical management and operational direction for the daily operation, activities and personnel for the Pediatric Intensive Care Unit (PICU). Their duties may include scheduling and staffing, documentation, performance improvement and budgetary compliance along with staff development, physician relationships, quality initiatives, program development, and system-wide success.

NURSE MANAGER-REHAB SERVICES

Provides clinical management and operational direction for the daily operation, activities and personnel for Rehab Services. Their duties may include scheduling and staffing, documentation, performance improvement and budgetary compliance along with staff development, physician relationships, quality initiatives, program development, and system-wide success.

NURSE MANAGER–RESPIRATORY INTENSIVE CARE UNIT

Provides clinical management and operational direction for the daily operation, activities and personnel for the Respiratory Intensive Care Unit (RICU). Their duties may include scheduling and staffing, documentation, performance improvement and budgetary compliance along with staff development, physician relationships, quality initiatives, program development, and system-wide success.

NURSE MANAGER-SUPPORT SERVICES

Provides clinical management and operational direction for the daily operation, activities and personnel for Support Services. Their duties may include scheduling and staffing, documentation, performance improvement and budgetary compliance along with staff development, physician relationships, quality initiatives, program development, and system-wide success.

NURSE MANAGER-SURGICAL SERVICES

Provides clinical management and operational direction for the daily opertion, activities and personnel for Surgical Services. Their duties may include scheduling and staffing, documentation, performance improvement and budgetary compliance along with staff development, physician relationships, quality initiatives, program development, and system-wide success.

NURSE MANAGER-TELEMETRY

Provides clinical management and operational direction for the daily operation, activities and personnel for the Telemetry Unit. Their duties may include scheduling and staffing, documentation, performance improvement and budgetary compliance along with staff development, physician relationships, quality initiatives, program development, and system-wide success.

NURSE MIDWIFE

Provides comprehensive primary health care to a select population of essentially healthy women under the supervision of a physician. Participates in the care of women with medical complications in collaboration with the OB/GYN physician. Provides comprehensive primary health care to a select population of essentially healthy women under the supervision of a physician. Participates in the care of women with medical complications in collaboration with the OB/GYN physician.

NURSE NAVIGATOR

Provides patient preparedness for treatment through education and psychosocial support. They facilitate interaction between patients and their physicians, provide logistical support, secure referrals, and assist with financial and insurance issues. Successful care coordination programs have been developed for many chronic diseases, including heart disease and diabetes and after a cancer diagnosis and through treatment.

NURSE PRACTITIONER (NP)

An advanced practice registered nurse (APRN) who has completed graduate-level education (earned a Master of Nursing or Doctor of Nursing Practice degree). A NP can diagnose diseases and provide appropriate treatment including prescribing medications. They can serve as primary care providers (PCPs) or work within a medical practice. An NP focuses on medical conditions and wellness, prevention, and quality of life.

NURSE RECRUITER

Responsible for recruiting qualified nursing applicants for all areas of the hospital. Plans advertisements, attends job fairs and coordinates in-house recruiting efforts. Conducts the initial interviews and recommends candidates to management.

NURSING ASSISTANT (NA)

An individual who gives basic nursing care under the supervision of a registered nurse or a licensed vocational nurse. NAs are also called nurse's aides, nursing attendants, health care assistants or orderlies. Responsible for a wide range of patient care tasks performed under the direction of a registered nurse. Tasks include activities of daily living and basic nursing care.

NURSING SUPERVISOR

An RN that supervises and coordinates all of the activities of personnel assigned to a specific shift.

OB/GYN CHIEF

A licensed physician that oversees the obstetric and gynecologic unit within a hospital.

OB/GYN CLINICAL NURSE

Provides nursing care to patients within the obstetrical and gynecological departments. Performs total patient care in the labor and delivery and postpartum unit.

OBSTETRICIAN/GYNECOLOGIST

A licensed physician that diagnoses, treats and helps prevent diseases of the reproductive tract of women and problems with childbirth. This physician often serves as the primary care physician for female patients.

OCCUPATIONAL THERAPIST (OT)

Responsible for organizing and conducting medically prescribed therapy treatment to individuals with developmental, physical, cognitive and/or emotional impairments, disabilities and/or handicaps, with the goal of helping the patient attain a maximum level of independence and performance. The therapist plans treatment programs within an interdisciplinary environment. This individual also is responsible for documentation and communication of all treatment information to appropriate parties.

OCCUPATIONAL THERAPIST ASSISTANT

An allied health professional who, under the direction of an occupational therapist, directs an individual's participation in selected tasks to restore, reinforce, and enhance their performance. They also help individuals re-learn skills and functions; correct disorders; and promote and maintain health.

OFFICE MANAGER-PHYSICIAN

Supervises the daily operation and administrative function of the physician office. Ensures the office is running smoothly by supervising office staff, hires, terminates, and trains employees, and oversees the billing portion of the office.

OMBUDSMAN

An official appointed to investigate a patient's complaint against the hospital.

ONCOLOGIST

A physician that specializes in the treatment of cancer.

ONCOLOGY DATA COORDINATOR

Coordinates the Oncology Data Registry and oncology data management program in accordance with established standards, policies, and regulations related to cancer surveillance and hospital cancer programs.

ONCOLOGY NURSE

Responsible for assessing, planning, implementing, and evaluating nursing care for patients in the hospitals Cancer Center or other designated area.

ONCOLOGY SERVICES DIRECTOR

Coordinates medical care as it relates to oncology program development and planning, quality, financial performance, and research.

ONCOLOGY SURGERY

The use of surgery to remove cancerous tumors or tissue.

OPERATING ROOM (OR) AID

Assists and supports the nurses and physicians in the delivery of surgical services through indirect patient care activities such as assisting in turning rooms over which includes bed cleaning, removing trash and emptying dirty linens; running errands, obtaining, moving and returning equipment, pharmacy orders and/or central supplies; inventories and stocks assigned areas and equipment and assists in the movement, positioning and transporting of patients.

OPERATING ROOM (OR) BUYER

Assures availability of surgical implants, specialty supplies and instruments for surgical cases. Ensure surgical supplies, instruments and implant expenses are controlled and patient billing is accurate. Ensures instrument and equipment repairs are tracked. Monitors par levels of required supplies and implants for turn rate and adjusts as required. Uses established systems and resources to provide excellent customer service including trouble shooting when problems occur and knows who to go to for help.

OPERATING ROOM (OR) SCHEDULER

The individual that schedules patients for surgery and schedules the surgeons, and assistants needed for the procedure by operating room. Distributes pre- and post-operative information to patients.

OPERATING ROOM (OR) SPECIALIST

This position replaces the manufacturer's sales rep in the OR. They assure availability of surgical implants, specialty supplies and instruments for surgical cases. Ensures surgical supplies, instruments and implant expenses are controlled and patient billing is accurate. Also ensures that instrument and equipment repairs are tracked. Monitors par levels of required supplies and implants for turn rate and adjusts as required. Uses established systems and resources to provide excellent customer service including trouble shooting when problems occur and knows who to go to for help.

OPERATING ROOM (OR) SURGICAL SERVICES MANAGER

The Manager of Surgical Services is directly responsible for the operation of the OR. Responsibilities include: scheduling; running the board, payroll, evaluations, disciplining staff, and reporting to the Director of Perioperative Services.

OPERATING ROOM (OR) TECH

Responsible for assisting with surgical procedures within the operating room.

OPHTHALMOLOGIST

A physician that specializes in the diagnosis and treatment of eye diseases and disorders such as cataracts and glaucoma and also prescribes corrective eyeglasses.

ORAL/MAXILLOFACIAL SURGEON

A physician that specializes in surgical correction of deformities, injuries and diseases of the mouth, teeth, jaws and facial structures.

ORAL SURGEON

A dentist that has specialized training in surgery of the mouth and jaw.

ORTHOPEDIC SURGEON

A physician that focuses on the preservation and restoration of the musculoskeletal system. Many orthopedic surgeons specialize in either a region of the body (such as the hand) or in a particular procedure (such as joint replacement).

ORTHOPEDIC SURGERY CHIEF

A licensed physician that oversees the division of the hospital pertaining to orthopedic surgery. Orthopedic surgery relates to the bones, joints and the musculoskeletal system (shoulders, knees and hips and related structures).

ORTHOPEDIC TECHNICIAN

Applies and adjusts plaster casts and assembles and attaches orthopedic traction equipment and devices as directed by a physician. Sets up bed traction units and inspects and adjusts bandages and equipment.

ORTHOPEDIST

Another name for a physician that is an orthopedic surgeon.

OTOLARYNGOLOGIST

A physician that specializes in treatment of conditions of the ears, neck and throat. Their expertise includes head and facial reconstructive and plastic surgery.

OTOLARYNGOLOGIC SURGEON

Otolaryngologic surgeons are more commonly known as ear, nose and throat (ENT) specialists. They diagnose and treat problems including ear diseases, sinusitis, tonsillitis and snoring. They also treat cancers of the skin, larynx, mouth and throat. ENT specialists also handle trauma patients and perform cosmetic surgeries.

PAIN MEDICINE SPECIALIST

A physician that focuses on the evaluation and management of people with acute and chronic pain. Pain management physicians come from many diverse medical specialties such as: Anesthesiology, Neurosurgery, Neurology, Physical Medicine and Rehabilitation, Psychiatry, Internal Medicine, Family Practice and other disciplines.

PAINTER

The individual assigned to paint or re-paint areas of the hospital.

PARKING LOT ATTENDANT

Parks and retrieves cars from the parking lot or parking structure for those wanting valet service. Also called Valet.

PATHOLOGIST

A physician that diagnoses and monitors disease through the microscopic examination of tissue specimens, cells, body fluids and secretions. Their work is essential in making diagnoses, prognoses and establishing treatment plans.

PATHOLOGY ASSISTANT

Coordinates the receiving, processing and gross description of all patient tissue specimens sent to the lab for diagnostic evaluation and postmortem examinations by a histopathologist.

PATIENT ACCESS REPRESENTATIVE

Accountable for greeting and directing patients and visitors. Also called Auxiliary, Hospital Greeter or Volunteer.

PATIENT ACCOUNT REPRESENTATIVE

The Patient Account Representative is responsible for processing billing and collection assignments in accordance with policies and procedures. Specific duties may include managing and reconciling accounts, along with updating and documenting financial data.

PATIENT CARE MANAGER (PCM)

A registered nurse who supervises a nursing unit.

PATIENT FINANCIAL SERVICE REPRESENTATIVE

Coordinates and facilitates patient billing and collection activities in one or more assigned areas of billing, payment posting, collections, payor claims research, and other accounts receivable work.

PATIENT FINANCIAL COUNSELOR-ADMITTING

Obtains complex financial information regarding patients from various sources, notifies insurance companies and assists with obtaining insurance authorizations. Handles and tracks payments, special package plan agreements, financial assistance paperwork, ability to obtain Medicaid applications, alternative financing, and verifies coverage from other third party payers in a variety of hospital settings. Utilizes effective collection activities to secure payment for balances on inpatient and outpatient accounts.

PATIENT MANAGEMENT COORDINATOR

Coordinates the flow of patients through the facility by assigning patients to beds based on bed availability, care needed, and patient type. Also arranges for patient transfers or admission. May act as a liaison with scheduling to ensure adequate levels of staff on duty.

PATIENT REGISTRATION REPRESENTATIVE

Collects data on new patients, inputs financial and demographic information into the computer system and collects co-pays if appropriate.

PATIENT SERVICE ASSISTANT (PSA)

Transports patients and assist nurses in meeting patients' personal needs.

PATIENT SERVICE COORDINATOR (PSC)

Answers telephone calls to the hospital unit and responds when a patient or family member presses the "call" button in the room. Also called Unit Secretaries.

PATIENT SERVICES SUPERVISOR

Oversees and coordinates the daily operations and activities for the central business unit or patient accounting department.

PATIENT TRANSPORT DISPATCHER

Provides efficient and timely coordination of transport services within the hospital.

PATIENT TRANSPORTER

Provides prompt, courteous transportation services to patients and visitors.

PAYROLL SUPERVISOR

Supervises the payment to all employees for routine pay, shift differentials, holidays, overtime and any additional compensation provided in accordance with their job description.

PAYROLL CLERK

Inputs data into the computerized payroll system, balances the payroll run and produces the federal, state and local tax payments and answers employee payroll questions.

PEDIATRIC NURSE

Provides care for children in all aspects of health care. Pediatric nurses practice in a variety of settings which include hospitals, clinics, schools, and in the home.

PEDIATRIC NURSE PRACTITIONER (PNP)

A nurse with advanced training in the nursing care of infants and children.

PEDIATRIC SURGEON

Examines, diagnoses, and surgically treats children from the newborn stage through late adolescence. Treats a wide variety of problems children may have, which may include appendicitis, hernias, cancer, or a serious congenital anomaly.

PEDIATRICIAN

Diagnoses, treats and helps prevent diseases and injuries of children.

PERFORMANCE IMPROVEMENT SPECIALIST

Plans, coordinates and manages assigned projects which support the hospital's Performance Improvement and Quality, Patient Safety and Customer Service Initiatives. Collaborates with all relevant internal and external staff to ensure that assigned projects meet relevant accreditation standards and requirements, and that all work is coordinated to accomplish goals in the most cost-effective, valid and accurate way possible.

PERFUSIONIST

Operates the heart and lung machine during procedures that require cardiovascular and/or cardiopulmonary bypass.

PERINATOLOGIST

A physician that provides specialized care to pregnant women and their fetuses.

PERIODIC AUTOMATIC REPLENISHMENT (PAR) DISTRIBUTION TECH

Responsible for the inventory, picking and replenishment of supplies, on the nursing floors, intensive care units and other designated areas and for the removal of outdated supplies.

PERIOPERATIVE NURSE

Operating room nurses are now referred to as Perioperative Registered Nurses to more accurately reflect their duties immediately before, during, and after surgery. These nurses provide surgical patient care by assessing, planning, and implementing the nursing care patients receive before, during and after surgery. These activities include patient assessment, creating and maintaining a sterile and safe surgical environment, pre- and post-operative patient education, monitoring the patient's physical and emotional well-being, and integrating and coordinating patient care throughout the surgical care continuum.

PHARMACIST (CLINICAL)

Oversees the daily activities of the medication use process, provides comprehensive contemporary pharmacy services (compounding/dispensing prescribed medications for patient care) and performs the duties of a registered pharmacist as defined by the State Board of Pharmacy and the hospital. Also serves as a resource to other healthcare professionals including pharmacy students and residents. Consults with Nursing, Medical Staff and patients regarding medications, orders, drug and pharmaceutical detail, patient reactions, errors and complaints and/or the patients' caregivers. Pharmacists who have completed a four-year professional curriculum along with a minimum of 1,740 hours of clinical experience earn the Doctor of Pharmacy (PharmD) degree.

PHARMACY ASSISTANT/AIDE

Assists the pharmacist in filing all orders, stocks shelves, checks prices and maintains proper inventory.

PHARMACY TECHNICIAN

Under supervision fills routine orders for unit doses and prepackaged pharmaceuticals and the delivery of medications. They serve as a liaison to assist in the appropriate and timely delivery of information and pharmaceutical products.

PHLEBOTOMIST

Draws blood for various medical tests and sends it to the laboratory.

PHYSICIAN EXTENDER

Another name for nurse practitioner or physician assistant. They perform medical activities in lieu of a physician.

PHYSICAL THERAPIST (PT)

Responsible for organizing and conducting medically prescribed therapy treatment to individuals with developmental, physical, cognitive and/or emotional impairments, disabilities and/or handicaps, with the goal of helping the patient attain a maximum level of independence and performance. The Therapist plans treatment programs within an interdisciplinary environment. This individual also is responsible for documentation and communication of all treatment information to appropriate parties.

PHYSICAL THERAPY ASSISTANT (PTA)

The Physical Therapy Assistant is responsible for a wide range of therapy treatment programs, performed under the guidance of the department director or physical therapists.

PHYSICIAN

An individual who has received a doctor of allopathy degree (M.D.) or doctor of osteopathy degree (D.O) and is currently licensed to practice medicine in the state.

PHYSICIAN ASSISTANT (PA)

Depending on state laws, physician assistants (PAs) generally have a formal relationship with a physician supervisor. The physician must be licensed within the state in which the PA is working, but does not have to work at the same location. Supervision can be in person or via telecommunications or consultation. Many PAs practice alone in remote or underserved areas in satellite clinics. Physician assistants conduct physical exams, diagnose and treat illnesses, order and interpret tests, counsel on preventive health care, assist in surgery, give medical orders, and write prescriptions. PAs work in hospitals, clinics, and other types of health facilities and exercise autonomy in medical decision making as determined by the supervising physician.

PHYSICIAN EXTENDER

A highly skilled healthcare practitioner who works under the general supervision of a licensed physician to provide patient care services. They can perform responsibilities delegated to them by a physician in the diagnostic and therapeutic management of patients. Examples are Physician Assistants (PA) and Certified Registered Nurse Practitioners (CRNP).

PHYSICIAN OFFICE MANAGER

Responsible for overseeing the day-to-day operations of a physician practice at either one or multiple sites including employee scheduling and development, Information Systems, physician scheduling, maintenance of medical records and files, quality management, office billing and collections, purchasing supplies and managing expenses. Also called a Medical Office Manager.

PHYSICIAN OFFICE REPRESENTATIVE

Assists with patient registration and accepts payments for physician/clinic services. Also schedules, confirms, and verifies patient appointments and insurance information and receives and directs phone calls, patients, and other visitors.

PHYSICIAN RECRUITER

Responsible for all physician recruitment and their on-boarding process. Recruits qualified physicians and develops the strategic plan to recruit physicians to meet the needs of the hospital. Performs the initial interviews to determine a candidate's suitability to the position and a facility.

PICTURE ARCHIVING AND COMMUNICATION SYSTEM MANAGER (PACS)

Responsible for the short and long term storage, retrieval, management, distribution and presentation of medical images. This system allows a hospital to capture, store, view and share all types of images internally and externally.

PLANT MECHANIC

Operates and assists in the proper maintenance and repairs of the hospital power plant, utilities, equipment and systems. They maintain and repair steam and hot water boilers, centrifugal and reciprocating chillers, and cooling towers. They ensure all pumped systems including: chilled water, condensate water, hot and cold water, heating hot water, condensate, sewage ejector, medical air, vacuum, mechanical air, and fuel oil are working properly. They also assist in the operating of the emergency generator system, fire monitoring and control systems.

PLASTIC RECONSTRUCTIVE SURGEON

A licensed physician that examines, diagnoses, and surgically treats patients that have abnormal structures of the body caused by congenital defects, developmental abnormalities, trauma, infection, tumors, or disease. Performs surgery to improve functions and to approximate a normal appearance.

PLASTIC SURGEON

Surgeons that repair, restore and replace physical defects of form or function of the craniofacial structures, the oropharynx, the upper and lower limbs, the breast and the external genitalia. This includes aesthetic surgery of these structures and undesirable form. They are skilled in the management of complex wounds and implantable materials. Also called Cosmetic or Reconstructive Surgeons.

PLUMBER

Performs installation, repair, assembly and maintenance of water, sewage, drainage, air, gas and vacuum systems and related equipment and facilities in accordance with pertinent state and local codes.

PODIATRIST

An individual who has received a doctor of podiatric medicine (D.P.M.) degree and who is fully licensed to practice podiatry in the state. They diagnose and treat conditions of the foot, ankle, and related structures of the leg.

POPULATION HEALTH NURSE

Provides care coordination across the continuum of care through telephonic population and disease management. Identifies, plans, coordinates, implements, monitors and evaluates appropriate cost-effective health care and utilization of services for patients to optimize patient function and well-being. This position provides for optimal outcomes through collaboration with the client, the family, the physician, health plan and other members of the healthcare team.

POST-ANESTHESIA CARE UNIT (PACU) NURSE

Provides nursing care to patients while they are in the post anesthesia care unit.

POWER PLANT OPERATOR

Maintains and ensures the proper operation of the hospitals operations to include: HVAC, medical air & vacuum systems, boiler plant equipment and related systems. Performs a wide range of advance technical preventive maintenance and repairs for assigned facility and/or department to include plumbing and electrical.

PRACTICE ADMINISTRATOR

The individual that takes care of the daily activities of a medical facility. They ensure the facility is properly staffed by recruiting physicians, nurses, medical assistants, and non-medical staff. They prepare the budget for staffing and training and negotiate contracts with medical supply companies and pharmaceutical companies to ensure that their facility has all of the necessary supplies.

PRIMARY CARE PHYSICIAN (PCP)

A physician who has the majority of their practice devoted to internal medicine, family/general practice and pediatrics. They often treat a variety of health problems across all patient age groups and frequently serve as the patient's first point of contact with the health care system

PROCUREMENT CATEGORY MANAGER

Leads the development and execution of key spend categories and strategic spend initiatives (e.g. supplier research, spend analytics, supplier due diligence, RFQ / RFP initiatives, negotiations, cost-out projects, LEAN initiatives) for a specific department or function of the hospital .i.e. surgery, laboratory etc. Also performs supplier management, supplier performance/development and inventory management initiatives. Example: a Perioperative Materials Buyer.

PROGRAM DIRECTOR – BEHAVIORAL HEALTH/PSYCHIATRY

An individual with the preparation, experience and expertise (usually masters or doctoral level) to manage the complex regulatory and clinical environment of a behavioral health inpatient program. Generally, this mid-level executive is responsible for overall unit operations and compliance with administrative responsibly for all disciplines and program quality, financial performance, etc.

PROJECT MANAGER

Plans, directs, coordinates and delivers project activities through the entire project life cycle that are major, complex and business critical. Ensures project objectives are completed on time, on budget, and in conformance to the hospital's standards.

PSYCHIATRIC/CLINICAL SOCIAL WORKERS

Usually, independently licensed social workers in their state of practice. Provides overall coordination of patient dispositions and transitions to lower levels of care based upon a psycho-social evaluation. Social Workers manage patient interactions and linkages with outside stakeholders, family members and service providers including outpatient programs, mental health centers, substance abuse providers, etc. Social workers also often coordinate payment and benefit eligibility services to ensure patients maintain or obtain access to care provided by third party payers or governmental programs. Social workers also provide individual and group psychotherapy where appropriate to individuals in addition to crisis intervention and ongoing care planning.

PSYCHIATRIC NURSE

Provides age-sensitive, professional patient care on the psychiatric unit as prescribed by the physician and/or needed by the patient including treatment planning and coordination, medication monitoring, group therapy, medication education, consultation and evaluations for emergency room patients or to provide crisis management evaluations for patients on other units of the hospital. Is experienced and skilled in physical and verbal crisis intervention techniques. Also called Behavioral Health Nurse.

PSYCHIATRIST

A licensed physician that diagnoses, treats and help prevents diseases of the mind. Serves as the primary clinical leader for inpatient psychiatric programs, directing treatment planning, treatment teams, determining length of stay, patient's risk level, legal status and suitability for transition to lower levels of care. Psychiatrists are MD's or DO's and are generally board certified in general, adult, geriatric or child & adolescent psychiatry.

PSYCHOLOGIST (PsyD)

An individual with a doctoral degree in psychology or a doctoral degree deemed equivalent by the State Board of Psychology and who is currently licensed to practice psychology. Generally psychologists provide neuropsychological testing to patients on inpatient units, but some may also provide forensic services and testimony in lieu of treating psychiatrists for civil detention hearings, competency proceedings, guardianship hearings, etc.

PULMONARY FUNCTION TECHNICIAN

Primarily performs diagnostic tests. These tests can include spirometry, diffusion testing, lung volumes, airway resistance, respiratory muscle forces, bronchial provocation testing and other tests that a doctor orders. They must also be able to calibrate, clean and maintain diagnostic equipment and recognize when equipment malfunctions. They may also work under the supervision of a doctor or nurse to deliver respiratory care services to patients in hospitals or other health care settings. They also perform tests on patients to assess potential pulmonary conditions. Some doctors ask pulmonary function technologists to also help treat patients who have a variety of cardiopulmonary disorders or other respiratory problems.

PULMONARY REHABILITATION TECHNICIAN

Works with a multidisciplinary team providing a structured set of services to patients two or three times per week for six to twelve weeks. This involves exercise training under the supervision of a healthcare professional, education about self-management strategies, nutrition, teaching the patient to partner with his or her doctor, and how the patient can apply what they learn at home.

PULMONOLOGIST

A physician that specializes in the diagnosis and treatment of diseases of the lungs and respiratory system. This includes diagnosis and treating lung cancer, pneumonia, asthma, pleurisy, sleep disorders and emphysema as well as others.

PURCHASED SERVICES ADMINISTRATOR

Supports the consistent delivery of Purchased Service contracts within a hospital or healthcare system. Requires a high level of professional knowledge in the preparation of RFPs/RFQs/RFIs, contracts, negotiation techniques, trends in healthcare, vendor management, and financial analysis to include in-source versus outsource review and cost-benefit analysis. Success is measured by meeting annual savings targets set annually by the department leadership.

PURCHASING AGENT-BUYER

Purchases supplies, capital equipment and purchased services to ensure an uninterrupted flow of goods at prices consistent with hospital standards for quantity, quality, safety and efficiency. Ensures that all efforts are exhausted to obtain quality product or service, on-time and at the best price. Also called a Purchasing Buyer or Strategic Procurement Buyer.

PURCHASING MANAGER

Responsible for the purchasing of all supplies, equipment, and services for the hospital or health System. Manages and ensures contract compliance. Plans, establishes and implements goals, objectives, policies, and procedures for the department. Directs the activities of the buyers, secretarial, and clinical staff toward providing the health system with the highest value equipment, purchase agreements and services.

QUALITY ASSURANCE DIRECTOR

Manages quality issues within the hospital or healthcare system. Investigates complaints, ensures that hospital services are of the highest quality.

Radiation Oncologist

A physician who specializes in treating cancer through radiation therapies and methods. Radiation therapy involves various kinds of radiation treatment techniques. The most common types of radiation therapy are 3-D treatment planning, external beam radiation, IMRT, stereotactic radiosurgery, prostate seed implants, brachytherapy and concurrent chemotherapy and radiation therapy. The oncologist selects the most effective radiation technique, for each particular patient, to destroy abnormal (cancer) cells while sparing the normal surrounding tissue. Radiation therapy is used on most types of cancers including breast cancer, lung cancer, prostate cancer, skin cancer, brain tumors and others.

Radiation Physicist

Consults with other members of the radiation oncology team and often assists with designing a treatment process. Before a treatment plan begins, the physicist is responsible for conducting quality assurance checks to ensure that of all parameters of the treatment have been correctly transferred to the machine and are correct for all treatment fields and that the plan is in accordance with the dose prescribed. At some hospitals, the physicist is responsible for education and training of the radiation oncology residents, radiology residents, Dosimetrists, nurses, and radiation therapists on the subject of radiation physics and radiobiology. Ensures quality radiation care and adherence to radiation standards are maintained throughout the planning and treatment process.

Radiation Therapist

Administers radiation treatment to patients via a machine called a linear accelerator. These devices project high-energy photon, electrons or protons at targeted cancer cells to shrink and eliminate cancerous tumors. As these particles collide with human tissue, they can shrink and eliminate cancerous tumors. During the treatment they keep detailed records of their patients' treatments such as the dose of radiation used for each treatment, the total amount of radiation used to date, the area treated, and the patient's reactions. Radiation oncologists and Dosimetrists review these records to ensure that the treatment plan is working, to monitor the amount of radiation exposure that the patient has received, and to keep side effects to a minimum.

Radiologist

A physician that uses radiation for the diagnosis and treatment of disease. This includes imaging diagnostic tests, including ultrasound, X-ray, CT, MRI, and PET. They also reads the images produced and issue a written report.

Radiologist-Interventional

A sub-specialty of Radiology that uses fluoroscopy, computerized axial tomography and ultrasound.

Radiology Technician/Technologist

Operates the X-ray equipment to make radiographs of various parts of the body. Specific duties includes properly positioning patients for procedures and providing radiation protection to patients and staff. This individual also is responsible for the proper development and storage of films, and may perform EKG testing and Holter monitor procedures.

Receptionist

Responsible for answering the telephone, greeting patients and visitors and scheduling appointments. These personnel typically work in hospitals, physician and dental offices and out-patient centers.

Rehab Care Nurse

Provides nursing care to patients within the rehabilitation care unit.

Rehab Technician

Assists members of the rehabilitation services team in providing patient care as established in the patient's treatment plan.

Referring Physician

A physician (usually a primary care physician) who provides a referral to a specialist.

Registered Nurse (RN)

A caregiver who has graduated from a college of nursing or other school of nursing and has passed a national licensing exam.

Reproductive Endocrinologist

This is a subspecialty within obstetrics and gynecology. Reproductive endocrinologists handle complex medical issues, involving hormonal imbalances in the reproductive system, such as infertility and recurrent miscarriages

REIMBURSEMENT MANAGER

Complete Medicare and Medicaid cost reports to obtain appropriate reimbursement in full compliance to federal and state regulations and the hospital's policies and procedures. Oversee the monthly close process to ensure the proper statement of governmental contractuals in accordance with hospital policies and procedures.

RESEARCH NURSE

Nurses that perform clinical and basic research.

RESIDENT

A licensed physician who takes part in advanced, supervised training. They participate in the patients care under the direction of an attending physician. Formerly, the first year after graduation was referred to as an "internship" and thereafter, as "residency." The years are now referred to as post-graduate years (PGY) I -V. (see PGY I, II, III, IV and V). Also called a House Physician.

RESOURCE SPECIALIST

Responsible for answering incoming and making outbound calls in a call center that assists consumers with physician referrals, educational classes and program registrations or outpatient visits. Schedules appointments for employed physician practices and makes outbound calls as needed for satisfaction surveys, class payment follow-ups or other information gathering or outreach needs.

RESPIRATORY CARE/THERAPY-NAVIGATOR

For patients with pulmonary disorders they provide preparedness for treatment after discharge through education and psychosocial support. This typically involves instructing and training patients on the proper use of CPAP, BIPAP, and other equipment; airway clearance methods; pacing and breathing exercises; smoking cessation; and all aspects of symptom management. They also assist discharge planners with respiratory equipment orders for discharge and work with MDs, RNs, and other hospital staff to coordinate the patient's care. They refer patients to outpatient services when appropriate and they provide training to home health and SNF agencies that receive patients. They also make follow-up calls to patients to ensure follow through with their plan of care after discharge and to encourage adherence to therapy and physician recommendations.

RESPIRATORY THERAPIST (RT)

A caregiver who has graduated from a college of respiratory care and has passed a licensing exam administered by the National Board for Respiratory Care. Responsible for a wide range of patient care tasks for those with respiratory disease and/or illness. Specific duties may include preparing, running and logging routine ECG and rhythm strips; preparing and administering oxygen therapy and aerosol modalities; interpreting and reporting vital signs and pulse oximetry; performing postural drainage and percussion; performing ventilator monitoring checks and changing ventilator circuits. This position frequently consults with physicians, while providing consultation instruction and/or technical direction of medical, nursing and other staff members.

REVENUE INTEGRITY MANAGER

Responsible for coordination and support for services throughout the revenue cycle and acts as an expert consultant to management on regulatory payer updates and issues, charge audit, clinical documentation, billing compliance, RACs, and payer credentialing. Manages and/or coordinates processes within the revenue cycle including periodic audits, training and corrective action plans. Manages department financials and staff.

RHEUMATOLOGIST

A physician that treat diseases of the joints, muscles, bones and tendons. They handle conditions including arthritis, back pain, muscle strains, athletic injuries and collagen diseases. They often work closely with specialists such as orthopedic surgeons and physical therapists.

RISK MANAGEMENT COORDINATOR

Assists the Director of Risk Management in coordinating hospital-wide risk management and insurance activities which include developing and maintaining systems for risk identification; investigation, prevention and reduction; managing claims against the medical center; managing, analyzing and distributing risk management data; conducting educational programs and providing consultative services on risk management issues.

RN-FIRST ASSISTANT

After completing extensive additional education and training to deliver direct surgical care, the RN First Assistant may directly assist the surgeon by controlling bleeding and by providing wound exposure and suturing during the actual procedure.

SAFETY DIRECTOR

Oversees all aspects of safety for patients, employees, etc. Provides leadership and expertise in the delivery of safe patient care. Integrates the information obtained from the reporting of adverse events, near misses and concerns related to clinical risk, patient complaints or other safety issues. Also develops responsive programs that enhance an organizational culture that supports patient safety.

SCHEDULING CLERK

Schedules all inpatient and outpatient procedures, admissions, pre-admissions for surgery patients and requests submitted by physicians and any other potential patient sources. Requests physician orders and insurance authorizations for tests and procedures ordered to ensure appropriate documentation is obtained prior to patient registration.

SCRUB TECH

Provides sterile instruments, prepares the patients for surgery by cleaning and shaving the skin, transfers the patient to the operating table, sterilizes the instruments, maintains the cleanliness of the operating room, and last, but not least, helps the surgical team "scrub in".

SECURITY DIRECTOR

The individual In charge of all security in and for the hospital.

SECURITY OFFICER

This position tours the facilities and grounds; assists with the welfare and safety of personnel and patients; investigates critical incidents; assists employees, patients and visitors; interfaces with emergency response agencies; secures doors; monitors parking and traffic control.

SERVICE LINE ADMINISTRATOR

This position is responsible for managing and growing the business service line while maintaining all appropriate clinical and quality guidelines for patient outcomes.

SLEEP LAB MEDICAL DIRECTOR

The licensed physician that oversees the sleep lab and specializes in the evaluation and treatment of sleep disorders.

SLEEP TECHNOLOGIST-TECHNICIAN

An allied health professional that works under the general supervision of a licensed physician to assist in the education, evaluation, treatment and follow-up of sleep disorder patients of all ages. They perform polysomnography and other tests used by a physician to diagnose and treat sleep disorders. Polysomnography includes the process of analyzing, monitoring, and recording physiologic data during sleep and wakefulness. During polysomnography this individual is responsible for attaching electrodes and monitors to patients who are participating in a sleep study, monitoring the patient throughout the sleep study, documenting observations and collecting data from various monitors and then reporting the information to a physician.

SOCIAL WORKER

An individual who is licensed by the state to practice social work. The social worker is responsible for patient care management across the continuum of care, as well as follow-up after discharge for a designated group of patients. Specific duties include counseling, education, supporting, and providing information to patients and families consistent with the principles of care and case management. Working in collaboration with registered Nurse Case Managers, physicians and other health care team members, the social worker is responsible for the ongoing assessment of patient needs and coordination and delivery of care with a significant focus on patient care outcomes. Some individuals have a bachelors in Social Work (BSW) while others have a Master's degree (MSW). Clinical Social Workers are always licensed so they often have a designation as Licensed Clinical Social Worker (LCSW) or a Licensed Master Social Work (LMSW).

SONOGRAPHER

A medical professional who operates ultrasound imaging devices to produce diagnostic images.

SONOLOGIST

A physician skilled in diagnostic ultrasound practice and interpretation.

SPEECH LANGUAGE PATHOLOGIST

Professionals who assess, diagnose and treat disorders related to speech, language, cognitive to communication, swallowing and fluency. They work with people who cannot produce sounds or produce them clearly, individuals who stutter, people with voice disorders, those that have trouble understanding or producing language and individuals with attention, memory and problem solving disorders and swallowing difficulties.

STAFF ACCOUNTANT

Responsible for the daily financial functions of the Accounting Department, including maintaining various spreadsheets, property and fixed asset files, journal entries, accounts payable support, and other projects as assigned.

STAFF NURSE

A generic term that describes a nurse that works within a hospital as a generalist or a specialist. Some nurses specialize in a specific type of care i.e. ICU or ED while others like to rotate to whichever department has an opening that meets their skill set.

STAFF PHYSICIAN

A fully credentialed physician who has completed training and is a member of the medical staff.

STAFFING COORDINATOR-NURSING ADMINISTRATION

Provides administrative support for clinical staffing, agency billing and documentation, scheduling and record keeping.

STERILE PROCESSING COORDINATOR

Coordinates the decontamination, correct assembly and sterile processing of instruments and equipment for the assigned area and monitors and maintains inventory and equipment records.

STERILE PROCESSING TECHNICIAN

Responsible for the proper care and handling of all general and specialty instruments including the cleaning, decontamination, instrument identification, assembly, packaging and distribution, and sterilization of surgical instrumentation for the assigned area.

STRATEGIC PROCUREMENT BUYER

Purchases supplies, capital equipment and purchased services to ensure an uninterrupted flow of goods at prices consistent with hospital standards for quantity, quality, safety and efficiency. Ensures that all efforts are exhausted to obtain quality product or service, on-time and at the best price. Also called a Purchasing Buyer or Strategic Procurement Buyer.

SUPPLY CONTRACT ANALYST

Manages the supplies and contracts, negotiates with suppliers, assures GPO compliance, supports Value Analysis and participates in relationship building with physicians. Also maintains the contract master, analyzes prices paid, and targets supplies for budget savings.

SUPPLY TECH

Responsible for the daily receipt of medical supplies, equipment, furniture, etc. with a 100% accuracy. Ensures the timely delivery of merchandise to customers. Coordinates the daily return of undelivered or refused goods to vendors. Acts as a liaison between the internal customers and the distribution team in addressing concerns.

SURGEON

A licensed physician that treats, diseases, injuries and deformities by invasive measures.

SURGERY CENTER DIRECTOR

Responsible for providing nursing and administrative direction for all aspects of the daily operations for the Surgery Center.

SURGERY CHIEF

A hospital leadership position occupied by a surgeon that oversees the day-to-day tasks and activities of the surgical services team. Responsible for directing the hospital's research, personnel, education programs and clinical care.

SURGICAL FIRST ASSISTANT (SFA)

The individual providing primary assistance to the main surgeon during a surgical procedure. The assistant may prepare and position the patient for surgery, assist in visualization of the operating field, provide hemostasis, harvest surgical grafts, perform closure of incisions, and apply various wound dressings. In addition to these intraoperative duties, surgical first assistants also perform pre- and post-operative activities to facilitate optimal patient care. Individuals who become certified by the National Surgical Assistant Association (NSAA) earn the Certified Surgical Assistant (CSA) credential.

SURGICAL INVENTORY SPECIALIST

Maintains the computer Inventory Control System (desktop and handheld) for the surgery area. Controls the ordering and restocking process of supplies and maintains and distributes stock. Communicates with the OR Buyer for reordering using established procedures. Prepares requisitions for the OR Manager to review and approve per policy. This position often has a dual role within Sterile Processing.

SURGICAL ONCOLOGIST

A surgeon that focuses on the surgical management of tumors, especially cancerous tumors.

SURGICAL SUPPORT TECH

Transports patients and lab specimens, assists with patient positioning and maintains patient rooms to ensure a sterile environment along with clerical support as required.

SURGICAL TECHNOLOGIST

Selects and places surgical instruments, supplies and equipment during surgery. Scrubs in to surgery and provides instruments, sutures, and other sterile supplies during the surgical procedure. Individuals who become certified by the National Board of Surgical Technology and Surgical Assisting (NBSTSA), earn the Certified Surgical Technologist (CST) credential.

SYSTEM CONFIGURATION ANALYST

Oversees, monitors and maintains information systems and databases within an assigned area. Duties often include producing and providing various statistical reports and data as well as identifying and recommending areas of improvement.

TAX ANALYST

Performs tax compliance and reporting for the hospital/system including the preparation of federal income tax returns, state and local tax reports.

TELE-HEALTH TRAINED-PHYSICIAN, RN, NURSE, PHYSICIAN ASSISTANT OR NURSE PRACTITIONER

An individual that is trained to diagnose, treat and consult with patients through virtual technology.

TELEMETRY MONITOR TECHNICIAN

Monitors patients on the Telemetry System and reports arrhythmias and monitor lead warnings to the nurse providing care for the patient.

TELEPHONE OPERATOR

Provides assistance and information to consumers, business associates, patients, physicians, in some cases physicians/offices, hospital staff, and the general public in response to requests and inquiries received by telephone.

THORACIC SURGEON

Surgeons that diagnose and treat conditions within the chest area such as lungs and esophagus but excluding the heart. They treat lung cancer, esophageal and tracheal conditions, airway conditions and chest injuries. Thoracic surgeons are often able to use minimally invasive procedures, making surgery easier for patients.

TRANSPLANT NURSE

Works in a variety of hospital locations and assists physicians in the transplantation of various body parts which often include liver, kidney, pancreas, small bowel, heart, and lungs.

TRANSPORT SPECIALIST-RESPIRATORY CARE

This position provides assessment and appropriate interventions to stabilize a patient for transport through the use of critical thinking skills. They collaborate with the control physician pertaining to the delivery of care.

TRAUMA NURSE

Trauma Nurses care for patients in an emergency or critical care setting. They often provide care for traumatic injuries such as for accident victims, gun-shot wounds, stabbings etc.

TRAUMA SURGEON

A surgeon that examines, diagnoses, and surgically treats critically injured patients.

TRANSPORTER

Provides transportation via wheelchairs, gurneys, and hospital beds for patients needing to be moved from one location to another within the hospital.

TRAVEL NURSE

Works for an agency that provides nurses to hospitals and other health care facilities across the country. Travel nurses usually get to choose which locations they are willing to travel to and are typically given assignments which last for 13 weeks or more.

TUMOR REGISTRAR

Identifies, registers, and maintains records of all inpatient and outpatient cancer patients by using a tumor registry data system. Analyzes data and releases information in adherence to established ethical standards.

ULTRASOUND TECHNOLOGIST

Operates the ultrasound equipment to obtain high quality ultrasound examinations of various body parts as ordered by the physician. Also prepares patients for the test, processes images and assists the physician as needed.

UNIT CLERK-UNIT SECRETARY

The Unit Clerk is responsible for a wide range of administrative activities, while contributing to the efficient operation of the healthcare unit and optimizing department personnel's time. Specific duties may include completing and updating all patient data in the patient chart record. This individual also provides centralized referral and control when stationed at the main desk.

UROLOGIST

A physician that specializes in the diagnosis and treatment of diseases of the urinary tracts in both men and women, and the genital organs of men. This includes cancer treatment, as well as treatment for infections, urinary and kidney stones, infertility, incontinence, impotence and prostrate issues.

UROLOGY CHIEF

The licensed physician that oversees the department that deals with diseases and disorders of the genitourinary tract in males and females and with the reproductive system in males.

UROLOGY NURSE

Works in physician offices, surgery and provides patient care in hospitals in such specialties as oncology, male infertility, male sexual dysfunction, kidney stones, incontinence, and pediatrics. Urology nurses may also participate in such urological surgeries as surgery for cancer, general urology, plastic, infertility, brachytherapy, lithotripsy, and pediatric surgery.

VALET

Parks and retrieve cars from the parking lot or parking structure for those wanting valet service. Also called Parking Lot Attendant.

VASCULAR SURGEON

A surgeon that specializes in the diagnosis, medical management, and surgical treatment of patients with diseases of the blood vessels outside the heart and brain.

VICE PRESIDENT OF ACADEMIC AFFAIRS

Responsible for providing oversight to the development, direction and coordination of all graduate medical education activities within the hospital. Also serves as the institutions resource and educator related to GME administrative, operation and accreditation issues.

VICE PRESIDENT OF COMMUNITY AND GOVERNMENTAL AFFAIRS

Responsible for the health system's marketing, public relations, physician relations and governmental affairs.

VICE PRESIDENT FINANCE

Responsible for the overall financial administration of the organization including general accounting, data processing and financial reporting in accordance with all facility policies and procedures. The job typically includes directing the treasury, budgeting, auditing and tax accounting and real estate activities. Also called the Chief Financial Officer.

VICE PRESIDENT HUMAN RESOURCES

Responsible for the hospital or health system's employment, employee relations, compensation, benefits, employee education, diversity, child care services, employee health and language services.

VICE PRESIDENT INFORMATION SERVICES

Responsible for the planning, implementation, and management of information technology and resources supporting the hospital or health system.

VICE PRESIDENT INTERNAL AUDIT

Performs a systematic, disciplined approach to evaluating and improving the effectiveness of risk management, internal controls and the governance of processes within the hospital/health system. Responsible for developing the annual work plan, including internal audits on compliance related matters. These activities include development and maintenance of systems, policies, and procedures designed to assist the organizations employees in meeting their legal, professional, and ethical responsibilities consistent with their mission, vision and values.

VICE PRESIDENT LEGAL AFFAIRS & GENERAL COUNSEL

Provides legal support to the hospital or health system's business operations, transactions with other providers and the Governing Board or Board of Trustees. Also oversees the legal work provided to the hospital or health care system by outside law firms.

VICE PRESIDENT MEDICAL AFFAIRS (VPMA)

A physician member (D.O. or M.D.) of the medical staff that works in partnership to strengthen the relationship between hospital administration and the medical staff. Responsible for planning, organizing and directing the medical staff services for the entire hospital or healthcare system. Assists the medical staff in formulating standards of care and strategic direction for quality and ensures positive medical staff relations. Works to align medical staff goals with those of the hospital or healthcare system and ensures compliance with all quality, legal, and regulatory requirements. Participates in recruitment, selection, and evaluation of employed physicians, nurse anesthetists and physician assistants. Also provides resource utilization across all departments and assists with service line development along with oversight and direction of the research program and Institutional Review Board as the Institutional Officer for the IRB.

VICE PRESIDENT PATIENT CARE SERVICES

Responsible for the operational, financial, clinical and personnel activities of all clinical services. Specific duties include directing nursing services for the facility and working collaboratively with other care providers to meet patient care needs. They participate in the development and implementation of programs and services, provide leadership related to federal, state and/or accreditation regulations and activities associated with the practice of nursing; and work with the members of the management, ancillary and care provider team to assure operational effectiveness, clinical excellence, physician, employee and staff satisfaction. Also called Chief Nursing Officer.

VICE PRESIDENT PATIENT EXPERIENCE-SERVICE EXCELLENCE

Acts as the champion dedicated to creating a culture that inspires and promotes an exceptional experience for patients and families as demonstrated by quality outcomes and a superior service orientation. They design integration strategies, which promote the optimal patient and customer experience for all constituents (patients, families, customers, physicians, employees) system-wide and acts as a leadership coach to strengthen and reinforce organizational values, culture and service and organizational excellence.

VICE PRESIDENT PATIENT FINANCIAL SERVICES

Provides operational and strategic leadership for all patient billing and collection functions. The Patient Financial Services department provides all billing services for the hospital's inpatient departments, outpatient services, and physician practices.

VICE PRESIDENT REVENUE CYCLE MANAGEMENT

Responsible for engaging in revenue cycle analysis, planning, budgeting and reporting to assist senior leaders across the hospital or health system in evaluating financial productivity and avenues for enhancement, including business development and revenue enhancement initiatives.

VICE PRESIDENT STRATEGY & BUSINESS DEVELOPMENT

Creates, administers and implements the business development functions of the hospital, its departments and various affiliates, and the strategic planning function for the designated market. As a member of the Executive Leadership Team, this individual leads these functions in accordance with established institutional long-range plans and objectives. This includes strategic long- and short-range plan development and service line development for the hospital.

VICE PRESIDENT-SUPPLY CHAIN MANAGEMENT

Provides strategic planning, direction and leadership for supply chain management operations at the enterprise level (all hospitals, clinics, system services etc.). Integrates all aspects of the supply chain management process throughout the enterprise and has overall accountability in meeting organizational objectives for supplies and non-labor services, the Value Analysis Program, centralized procurement, contract negotiation, inventory management (Just-in-Time, JIT), stockless and procedure/case based delivery), Group Purchasing Organization (GPO) relationships, Receiving, Storage, Distribution, Stock Replenishment and Asset Management for all supplies, services and equipment utilized by the enterprise. Prepares and manages budgets, manages/supervises staff and ensures quality services are provided through daily operations

VICE PRESIDENT TALENT ACQUISITION

This position leads, defines, designs, integrates and implements key Human Resource initiatives and strategies in the areas of talent acquisition to include executive, physician, clinical and non-clinical recruitment, mergers and acquisitions, sourcing and advertising, work force planning and outreach efforts.

VOLUNTEER COORDINATOR

The individual that recruits, interviews and coordinates the assignments of volunteers within the facility. The staff work at the reception desk and in the hospital gift shop. Many also deliver flowers to patient rooms and direct /take visitors to their desired location. Also called Auxiliary.

VOLUNTEER

Individuals that volunteer their time to work at the reception desk and in the hospital gift shop. Many also deliver flowers to patient rooms and direct or take visitors to their desired location. Also called Auxillary.

WEB DEVELOPER

Develops and maintains the hospital web site. Oversees a group of graphic designers to provide content updates and upgrades.

WOMEN'S HEALTH NURSE

These nurses practice in a variety of settings and participate in areas such as OB/GYN, mammography, reproductive health, and general women's health.

WOUND CARE NURSE

A nurse who specializes in wound management. These nurses can also care for ostomy sites, as well as the areas around feeding tubes, ports, and recent surgeries. Most work in a hospital setting or in skilled nursing facilities.

APPENDIX 1

ACRONYMS & MEDICAL INDUSTRY ABBREVIATIONS

The hospital is a fast-paced, specialized medical community where it's common to use acronyms and abbreviations to describe anything from a clinician's credentials, to metrics or a credentialing body. While it may make communication simple for hospital personnel, it can be confusing to company personnel who are selling to the hospital or healthcare facility and who may not be familiar with the medical terminology. Below is a list of common abbreviations used throughout the hospital and what they mean.

AAAI-American Academy of Allergy & Immunology

AACN- American Association of Colleges of Nursing

AACOM-American Association of Colleges of Osteopathic Medicine

AACN American Association for Critical Care Nurses

AAFP-American Academy of Family Physicians

AAMC-Association of American Medical Colleges

AAN-American Academy of Nursing

AANA- American Association of Nurse Anesthetists

AANN-American Association of Neurological Nurses

AAOS-American Academy of Orthopaedic Surgeons

AAOS-American Association of Orthopaedic Surgeons

AAP-American Academy of Pediatrics

AAPA-American Academy of Physician Assistants

AAPMR-American Academy of Physical Medicine & Rehabilitation

AARC-American Association of Respiratory Care

ABMS-American Board of Medical Specialties

ABN-Advanced Beneficiary Notice

ABS-American Board of Surgery

ACA-Affordable Care Act

AC-Ambulatory Care

ACCP-American College of Chest Physicians

ACEP- American College of Emergency Physicians

ACCME-Accreditation Council for Continuing Medical Education

ACEHP-Alliance for Continuing Education in the Health Professions

ACFAS - American College of Foot & Ankle Surgeons

ACGME-American College of Graduate Medical Education

ACHE- American Academy of Healthcare Executives

ACMPE-Association American College of Medical Practice Executives

ACMVU-Adjusted Case Mix Value Units

ACO-Accountable Care Organization

ACOG- American College of Obstetrics & Gynecology

ACP-American College of Physicians

ACR-American College of Radiology

ACS-American College of Surgeons

ADA-Americans with Disabilities Act

ADC-Average Daily Census

ADE-Adverse Drug Event

ADL-Activities of Daily Living

AHA-American Hospital Association

AHCA-American Health Care Association

AHP-Allied Health Professional

AHRMM-Association for Healthcare Resources and Materials Management

AHRQ-Agency for Health Care Policy and Research

ALOS-Average Length of Stay

AMA-American Medical Association

AMA-Against Medical Advice

AMC-Academic Medical Center

AMGA-American Medical Group Association

ANA-American Nursing Association

ANCC-American Nurses Credentialing Center

ANNC-American Nurses Credentialing Center

AOA-American Osteopathic Association

AOFAS - American Orthopaedic Foot & Ankle Society

AONE-American Organization of Nurse Executives

AOTA- American Occupational Therapy Association

AP-Accounts Payable

APA-American Psychiatric Association

APC-Ambulatory Payment Classification

APIC-Association for Professionals in Infection Control and Epidemiology

APMA-American Podiatric Medical Association

APN-Advanced Practical Nurse

APRN-Advanced Practice Registry Nurse

AR-Accounts Receivable

ARRA- American Recovery & Reinvestment Act

ARRT-American Registry of Radiologic Technologists

ASA-American Society of Anesthesiologists

ASC-Ambulatory Surgery Center

ASCA-American Surgery Center Association

ASHA- American Speech, Language & Hearing Association

ASHE-American Society for Healthcare Engineering

ASHP-American Society Health Systems Pharmacists

ASHRM-American Society for Healthcare Risk Management

ASSH- American Society for Surgery of the Hand

ATS-American Thoracic Society

AWP-Average Wholesaler Price

BBP-Blood Borne Pathogens

BiPAP- Bilateral Positive Airway Pressure

BMT-Blood and Marrow Transplantation

BSN-Bachelor Degree in Nursing

BScN-Bachelor Degree in Nursing

BSW-Bachelor Degree in Social Work

BUN-Blood Urea Nitrogen

BWC-Bureau of Workers Compensation

BY-Budget Year

CAF- Contract Administrative Fee

CAH-Critical Access Hospital

CAP-College of American Pathologists

CAT-Computerized Axial Tomography

CBC-Complete Blood Count

CBT-Cognitive Behavioral Therapy

CCLS –Certified Child Life Specialist

CCU-Critical Care Unit

CCU-Cardiac Care Unit

CDAO-Chief Data Analytics Officer

CEO-Chief Executive Officer

CER-Comparative Effectiveness Research

CFO-Chief Financial Officer (CFO)

CHAMPUS-Civilian Health and Medical program for the Uniformed Services

CHF-Congested Heart Failure

CHIP-Children's Health Insurance Program

CICU-Cardiac Intensive Care Unit

CIO-Chief Information Officer (CIO)

CIO-Chief Innovation Officer

CIO-Chief Investment Officer

CLIA'88-Clinical Laboratory Improvement Amendment of 1988

CLMA–Clinical Laboratory Managers Association

CME-Continuing Medical Education

CMI-Case Mix Index

CMO-Chief Marketing Officer

CMO-Chief Medical Officer

CMIO-Chief Medical Information Officer (CMIO)

CMS-Center for Medicare & Medicaid Services

CMSS-Council of Medical Specialty Services

CNA-Certified Nursing Assistant

CNM- Certified Nurse Midwife

CNO-Chief Nursing Officer

CNIO-Chief Nursing Informatics Officer

CNS-Clinical Nurse Specialist

COB-Coordination of Benefits

COBRA-Consolidated Omnibus Budget Reconciliation Act

CON-Certificate of Need

COO- Chief Operations Officer

Co-Pay- Co-payment

COPD-Chronic Obstructive Pulmonary Disease

CORF-Comprehensive Outpatient Rehabilitation Facility

COTA-Certified Occupational Therapy Assistants

CPAP- Continuous Positive Airway Pressure

CPB- Cardiopulmonary Bypass

CPEO-Chief Patient Experience Officer

CPOE-Computerized Physician Order Entry

CPHO-Chief Population Health Officer

CPR-Customary, Prevailing, and Reasonable (charges)

CPR-Cardiac Pulmonary Resuscitation

CPT-Current Procedural Terminology

CPT-Custom Procedure Tray

CQI-Continuous Quality Improvement

CRM- Customer Relationship Management

CRNA-Certified Registered Nurse Anesthetist

CSA-Certified First Assistant

CST- Certified Surgical Technologist

CSO-Chief Strategy Officer

CT-Computerized Tomographic Scanner

CTO-Chief Transformation Officer

CTRS-Certified Therapeutic Recreation Specialist

DCRS-Data Comparison Reporting System

DEA-Drug Enforcement Agency

DHHS-Department of Health & Human Services

DME-Durable Medical Equipment

DNR-Do Not Resuscitate

DO-Doctor of Osteopathy

DOA-Dead on Arrival

DOB-Date of Birth

DOS-Date of Service

DRG-Diagnosis Related Group

DSH-Disproportionate Share Hospital Payment

DSO-Days Sales Outstanding

DX-Diagnosis

ECG-Electrocardiogram

ECMO-Extracorporeal Membrane Oxygenation

ED-Emergency Department

EDI-Electronic Data Interchange

EEG-Electroencephalogram

EHR-Electronic Health Record

EIN- Employer Identification Number

EKG-Electrocardiogram

EMPI- Electronic Master Patient Index

EMR-Electronic Medical Record

EMS-Emergency Medical Services

EMT-Emergency Medical Technician

ENT–Ears, Nose and Throat

EOQ- Economic Order Quantity

EP- Electrophysiology

EPHI-Electronic Protected Health Information

EOB-Explanation of Benefits

EOMB-Explanation of Medical Benefits

ERP-Enterprise Resource Planning

ETT or ET Tube-Endotracheal Tube

EVA- Economic Value Added

FACP- Fellow American College of Chest Physician

FACS-Fellow American College of Surgeons

FAH-Federation of American Hospitals

FDA-Food & Drug Administration

FFS-Fee for Service

FFY-Federal Fiscal Year

FI-Fiscal Intermediary

FOB-Free On Board

FP-Family Practice

FP-For-Profit Hospital

FPL-Federal Poverty Level

FSED-Free-Standing ED

FSMB-Federation of State Medical Boards

FTE-Full-Time Equivalent

FY-Fiscal Year

GAAP-Generally Accepted Accounting Principles

GME-Graduate Medical Education

GPO-Group Purchasing Organization

GYN-Gynecologist

HAI-Healthcare Associated Infection

HBV-Hepatitis B Virus

HCFA- Health Care Financing Administration

HCUPQI-Healthcare Cost and Utilization Project Quality Indicators

HEOR- Health Economics & Outcomes Research

HFMA- Healthcare Financial Management Association

HHA-Home Health Agency

HHS-Health and Human Services

HIM-Health Information Management

HIMSS-Healthcare Information and Management Systems Society

HIPPA-Health Insurance Portability and Accountability Act

HIT-Health Information Technology

HITECH-Health Information Technology for Economic and Clinical Health

HIV-Human Immunodeficiency Virus

HL-7- Health Level 7

HMIS–Hospital Management Information System

HMO-Health Maintenance Organization

HOPD-Hospital outpatient department

HQA- Hospital Quality Alliance

HR-Human Resources

HSCA-Healthcare Supply Chain Association

IADL-Instrumental Activities of Daily Living

ICD 10 CM-International Classification of Diseases, Clinical Modification

ICN-Intermediate Care Nursery

ICP–Intracranial Pressure

ICU-Intensive Care Unit

IDS-Integrated Delivery System

IDE- Investigational Device Exemption

IFEC-Independent freestanding emergency centers

IHI-Institute for Healthcare Improvement

IOM-Institute of Medicine

IPA-Independent Practice Association

IPPS-Inpatient Prospective Payment System

IRB-Institutional Review Board

ITB-Invitation to Bid

IT-Information Technology

ITB- Invitation To Bid

IW- Injured Worker

JIT- Just In Time

KPI- Key Performance Indicator

LBW-Low Birth Weight

LCSW-Licensed Clinical Social Work

LDR-Labor, Delivery, and Recovery room

LDRP-Labor, Delivery, Recovery, Postpartum room

LMSW – Licensed Master Social Work

LOS-Length of Stay

LP-Lumbar Puncture

LPN-Licensed Practical Nurse

LTACH-Long-Term Acute Care Hospital

LTC-Long-Term Care

LWBS-Left Without Being Seen

MA-Medicare Advantage

MAC-Medicare Administrative Contractor

MCO-Managed Care Organization

MD-Doctor of Medicine

MEC-Medical Executive Committee

MGMA-ACPME-Medical Group
Management

MICU- Medical Intensive Care Unit

MRI-Magnetic Resonance Imaging

MS-DRG-Medicare Severity DRG System

MSW–Master of Social Work

NA-Nursing Assistant

NAHDO-National Association Health Data
Organizations

NAHTM- National Association of
Healthcare Transport Management

NAP-NAP-National Association of Pediatric
Nurse Associates/Practitioners

NASS- North American Spine Society

NB-Newborn

NBME-National Board Medical Examiners

NBSTSA-National Board of Surgical
Technology & Surgical Assistants

NCHS-National Center for Health Statistics

NCQA-National Committee for
Quality Assurance

NCSBN-National Council of State
Boards of Nursing

NFP–Not for Profit

NG Tube-Nasogastric Tube

NHLBI-National Heart, Lung &
Blood Institute

NICU-Neonatal Intensive Care Unit

NICU-Neurological Intensive Care Unit

NICU-Neuroscience Intensive Care Unit

NNP-Neonatal Nurse Practitioner

NP-Nurse Practitioner

NPI- National Provider Identifier

NPP-Non-Physician Practitioner

NPP-Notification of Privacy Practices

NPPB-National Practitioner Data Bank

NPSG-National Patient Safety Goals

NQF-National Quality Forum

NRHA–National Rural Health Association

NTE- Not to Exceed

OB-Obstetrician/Gynecologist

OB-GYN- Obstetrics & Gynecology

OIG-Office of Inspector General

ONC-Office of the Coordinator of Health
Information Technology

OPPS-Outpatient Prospective
Payment System

OR-Operating Room

OSHA-Occupational Safety and Health
Administration

OT-Occupational Therapy/Therapist

P &T-Pharmacy and
Therapeutics Committee

P4P-Pay for Performance

PA-Physician Assistant

PACS-Picture Archiving and Communication System

PACU-Post Anesthesia Care Unit

PAR-Periodic Automatic Replenishment

PCM-Patient Care Manager

PCMH-Patient Centered Medical Home

PCP-Primary Care Physician

PCPI-Physician Consortium for Performance Improvement

PCU-Progressive Care Unit

PDR- Physician Desk Reference

PEC-Pre-Existing Condition

PET-Positron Emission Tomography

PGY-Post Graduate Year

PharmD-Doctor of Pharmacy

PHI- Personal Health Information

PHI-Protected Health Information

PICC-Percutaneous Line/Percutaneous Central Catheter

PICU-Pediatric Intensive Care Unit

PM&R-Physical Medicine and Rehabilitation

PNP-Pediatric Nurse Practitioner

PO-Purchase Order

POD- Physician Owned Distributorship

POS- Point of Service

PPI-Physician Preference Item

PPO-Preferred Provider Organization

PPS-Prospective Payment System

PQRI-Physician Quality Reporting Initiative

PSA-Patient Service Assistant

PSC-Patient Service Coordinator

PsyD-Doctor of Psychology

PT-Physical Therapy

PT-Physical Therapist

PTA-Physical Therapy Assistant

QA-Quality Assurance

QALYs-Quality Adjusted Life Years

QI-Quality Improvement

QIOs-Quality Improvement Organizations

R & C- Reasonable and Customary Charge

RAC-Recovery Audit Contractor

RBRVS-Resource-Based Relative Value Scale

RC- Referral Coordinator

RCM-Revenue Cycle Management

RD–Registered Dietitian

RICE- Rest, Ice, Compression, and Elevation

RFI-Request for Information

RFP-Request for Proposal

RFID- Radio Frequency Identification

RFQ-Request for Quotation

RFx-Request for Solicitation

RN-Registered Nurse

ROI-Return on Investment

RPO- Recruitment Process Outsourcing Firm

RRT-Rapid Response Team

RRT-Registered Respiratory Therapist

RT-Respiratory Therapy

RT-Respiratory Therapist

RTW-Return to Work

RVU-Relative Value Unit

SaaS-Software–as-a-Service

SCCM-Society of Critical Care Medicine

SCHIP- State Chilidrens Health Insurance Program

SEO- Search Engine Optimization

SEM- Search Engine Marketing

SFA- Surgical First Assistant

SICU-Surgical Intensive Care Unit

SLP- Speech Language Therapist

SNF-Skilled Nursing Facility

SOW-Statement of Work

SPD-Sterile Processing Department

SSL-Secure Sockets Layer

SSO-Single Sign-On

TAT-Turn-around Time

TIN-Tax Identification Number

TCU-Transitional Care Unit

TPA- Third Party Administrator

TPN-Total Parenteral Nutrition

TQM-Total Quality Management

UB-04-Medicare Claim Form

UCR-Usual, Customary and Reasonable

UR-Utilization Review

VA-Veterans Administration

VAC- Value Analysis Committee

VBP-Value Based Purchasing

VPMA-Vice President of Medical Affairs

WHO-World Health Organization

WHPUOS-Worked Hours per Unit of Service

APPENDIX 2

Anatomical Orientation Terms

AXIAL

Refers to the head, neck and trunk. This is the main portion of the human body.

ANTERIOR

The front of the human body or toward the front of the structure

Example: The stomach is anterior to the spine.

CRANIAL

Toward the head or upper portion of the body or a structure; above.

DEEP

Internal. Away from the exterior surface.

Example: The heart is deep relative to the skin.

DISTAL

Further from the beginning or the origin of a body part or the point of attachment to a body part or the trunk of the body.

Example: The foot is distal to the knee.

INFERIOR

Toward the lower part of the human body or a structure, away from the head or below.

Example: The chin is inferior to the eyes.

LATERAL

Toward the left or right side of the body; away from the midline.

Example: The arms are lateral to the heart.

MEDIAL

In the middle of a structure or in the middle of the human body.

Example: The sternum is medial to the arms.

POSTERIOR

The back of the human body or toward the back of the structure

Example: The spine is posterior to the heart.

PRONE

Lying face down.

PROXIMAL

Closer to the beginning or the origin of a body part or the point of attachment to a body part to the trunk of the body.

Example: The knee is proximal to the foot.

SUPERFICIAL

Toward or at the body surface.

Example: The skin is superficial to the muscles and bones.

SUPERIOR

The upper part of the human body or a structure, toward the head; above

Example: The head is superior to the chest. The nose is superior to the mouth.

SUPINE

Lying face up.

APPENDIX 3

Healthcare Agencies & Organizations

ACCREDITATION COUNCIL FOR CONTINUING MEDICAL EDUCATION (ACCME)
The organization that identifies, develops and promotes standards for quality continuing medical education (CME) used by physicians to improve quality medical care for patients and their communities. It is a voluntary self-regulated system for accrediting CME providers and a peer-review process.

AGENCY FOR HEALTH CARE POLICY AND RESEARCH (AHRQ)
An organization whose mission is to support research designed to improve the outcomes and quality of health care, reduce its costs, address patient safety and medical errors, and broaden access to effective services.

ALLIANCE FOR CONTINUING EDUCATION IN THE HEALTH PROFESSIONS (ACEHP)
The organization that offers educational programs and services to educators and professionals working in hospitals and health systems, academic medical centers, medical specialty societies, medical education communication companies, the government, and the pharmaceutical, medical device and biotech industries to improve their knowledge, skills, and expertise to improve health outcomes.

AMBULATORY SURGERY CENTER ASSOCIATION (ASCA)
The national membership association that represents ambulatory surgery centers (ASCs) and provides advocacy and resources to assist ASCs in delivering high quality, cost-effective ambulatory surgery to all the patients they serve.

American Academy of Allergy & Immunology (AAAI)

A national professional organization whose members are allergists and immunologists, other medical specialists and allied health and related healthcare professionals. Each has a special interest in the research and treatment of allergic and immunologic diseases.

American Academy of Family Physicians (AAFP)

The national professional association of family doctors. They have four objectives: advocacy, practice enhancement, education and health of the public.

American Academy of Nursing (AAN)

A part of the American Nurses Association that honors their members for superior achievement in nursing practice, education and research.

American Academy of Orthopaedic Surgeons (AAOS)

The national professional organization that provides musculoskeletal education to orthopaedic surgeons and other interested parties through its annual meeting, CME courses, medical and scientific publications and electronic media materials.

American Association of Orthopaedic Surgeons (AAOS)

The national professional organization that participates in health policy and advocacy activities on behalf of musculoskeletal patients and the profession of orthopaedic surgery.

American Academy of Pediatrics (AAP)

A national professional membership organization of primary care pediatricians, pediatric medical sub-specialists and pediatric surgical specialists dedicated to the health, safety, and well-being of infants, children, adolescents and young adults.

American Academy of Physical Medicine & Rehabilitation (AAPMR)

A national professional organization whose physician members are specialists in physical medicine and rehabilitation (PM&R).

American Academy of Physician Assistants (AAPA)

The national professional organization of physician assistants.

AMERICAN ASSOCIATION OF COLLEGES OF OSTEOPATHIC MEDICINE (AACOM)

A non-profit organization that supports the colleges of osteopathic medicine within the U.S. and serves as their unifying voice for osteopathic medical education. They provide centralized services to its members such as data collection and analysis and they operate an online application service for prospective students applying to osteopathic medical schools. They are also active in advocacy at the federal government level.

AMERICAN ASSOCIATION OF CRITICAL-CARE NURSES (AACN)

The national organization of nurses working in critical care units.

AMERICAN ASSOCIATION OF NEUROLOGICAL NURSES (AANN)

The national professional organization of nurses that works with neurologically impaired patients. These nurses practice in a variety of settings such as multispecialty and neuroscience intensive care units, general neuroscience units, rehabilitation units, combination units, emergency and trauma departments and surgery.

AMERICAN ASSOCIATION OF NURSE ANESTHETISTS (AANA)

The national professional organization of nurse anesthetists. These advanced practice nurses are called Certified Registered Nurse Anesthetists (CRNAs) and they practice in every setting where anesthesia is available.

AMERICAN ASSOCIATION OF RESPIRATORY CARE (AARC)

The AARC is a professional membership association for respiratory care professionals and allied health specialists interested in cardiopulmonary care.

AMERICAN BOARD OF MEDICAL SPECIALTIES (ABMS)

An organization of medical specialty boards with shared goals and standards related to the certification of medical specialists. Certification includes initial specialty and subspecialty certification and maintenance of certification throughout the physician's career.

AMERICAN BOARD OF SURGERY (ABS)

An independent, nonprofit organization founded to assess the qualifications of physicians in the field of surgery. They offer primary board certification in general surgery and vascular surgery, and secondary certification in several related specialties.

AMERICAN COLLEGE OF CHEST PHYSICIANS (ACCP)

An international professional association whose mission is to advance the best patient outcomes by championing the prevention, diagnosis, and treatment of chest diseases through innovative chest medicine education, clinical research, and team-based care.

AMERICAN COLLEGE OF EMERGENCY PHYSICIANS (ACEP)

A national professional organization whose physician members are specialists in emergency medicine.

AMERICAN COLLEGE OF FOOT & ANKLE SURGEONS (ACFAS)

A professional society of foot and ankle surgeons that promotes the art and science of foot, ankle and related lower extremity surgery. They are also active in health policy and advocacy, education and professional development, research and publication.

AMERICAN COLLEGE OF GRADUATE MEDICAL EDUCATION (ACGME)

The non-profit organization responsible for accrediting all of the graduate medical training programs for physicians (MD or DO) in the U.S.

AMERICAN COLLEGE OF HEALTHCARE EXECUTIVES (ACHE)

An international professional association of healthcare executives whose mission is to be the premier professional society for improving healthcare delivery.

AMERICAN COLLEGE OF OBSTETRICS & GYNECOLOGY (ACOG)

A national professional organization whose physician members includes obstetricians and gynecologists.

AMERICAN COLLEGE OF PHYSICIANS (ACP)

A national professional organization whose physician members includes internists, internal medicine subspecialists, and medical students, residents, and fellows. They apply their knowledge and expertise to keep adults healthy and diagnose, treat, and provide care when patients are ill.

AMERICAN COLLEGE OF RADIOLOGY (ACR)

The principal organization of radiologists, radiation oncologists, and clinical medical physicists in the United States.

AMERICAN COLLEGE OF SURGEONS (ACS)

The national professional association of physicians that specialize in surgery. Members are considered fellows and they abbreviate their membership status in the American College of Surgeons by using the letters FACS (Fellow, American College of Surgeons).

AMERICAN HEALTH CARE ASSOCIATION (AHCA)

A non-profit federation of affiliated state health organizations, that represents non-profit and for-profit nursing facility, assisted living, developmentally-disabled, and subacute care providers that care for elderly and disabled individuals.

AMERICAN HOSPITAL ASSOCIATION (AHA)

The national organization that represents and serves all types of hospitals, health care networks and their patients and communities. AHA takes part in national health policy development, legislative and regulatory debates, and legal matters. AHA also provides education for health care leaders and is a source of information on health care issues and trends.

AMERICAN MEDICAL ASSOCIATION (AMA)

A nonprofit professional association of physicians and medical students in the United States, including all medical specialties. Its purpose is to establish and promote ethical, educational, and clinical standards for the medical profession and to serve as an advocate for the advancement of the profession. It also provides education for health care leaders and is a source of information on health care issues and trends.

AMERICAN MEDICAL GROUP ASSOCIATION (AMGA)

A non-profit trade association representing physician-owned, independent group practices; Integrated delivery systems; hospital-affiliated medical groups; Independent practice associations (IPAs); Academic and faculty practices; Accountable care organizations and high-performing health systems

They are a leading voice in advocating for efficient, team-based, and accountable care.

AMERICAN NURSES ASSOCIATION (ANA)

A national professional organization to advance and protect the profession of nursing. The ANA advances the nursing profession by fostering high standards of nursing practice, promoting the rights of nurses in the workplace, projecting a positive and realistic view of nursing, and by lobbying the Congress and regulatory agencies on health care issues affecting nurses and the public.

AMERICAN NURSES CREDENTIALING CENTER (ANCC)

As a subsidiary of the American Nurses Association (ANA), this organization promotes excellence in nursing and health care globally through a variety of educational materials and credentialing programs that recognizes individual nurses in specialty practice areas. They also recognize healthcare organizations that promote nursing excellence and quality patient outcomes while providing safe, positive work environments and they accredit healthcare organizations that provide and approve continuing nursing education.

AMERICAN OCCUPATIONAL THERAPY ASSOCIATION (AOTA)

The national professional association of occupational therapists, occupational therapy assistants and students studying occupational therapy.

AMERICAN ORGANIZATION OF NURSE EXECUTIVES (AONE)

An organization that is dedicated to providing leadership, professional development, advocacy and research to advance nursing practice and patient care. It also promotes nursing leadership excellence and shapes public policy for health care nationwide. AONE is a subsidiary of the American Hospital Association.

AMERICAN OSTEOPATHIC ASSOCIATION (AOA)

A national professional association organized into local and regional societies that represent osteopathic physicians in the United States.

AMERICAN ORTHOPAEDIC FOOT & ANKLE SOCIETY (AOFAS)

The national professional organization of orthopaedic surgeons that specializes in the care of patients with injuries, diseases, and other conditions of the foot and ankle. Their active members are certified by the American Board of Orthopaedic Surgery, American Osteopathic Board of Orthopedic Surgery or the Royal College of Physicians and Surgeons of Canada.

AMERICAN PODIATRIC MEDICAL ASSOCIATION (APMA)

A professional medical organization that represents podiatrists within the United States. They also accredit the nation's podiatric medical schools.

AMERICAN PSYCHIATRIC ASSOCIATION (APA)

A national professional organization whose physician members specialize in the diagnosis, treatment, prevention, and research of mental illnesses including substance abuse disorders. They ensure proper care and effective treatment for all individuals with mental disorders, including intellectual disability and substance abuse disorders.

AMERICAN REGISTRY OF RADIOLOGIC TECHNOLOGISTS (ARRT)

The credentialing organization for radiological technologists in the disciplines of medical imaging, interventional procedures, and radiation therapy. They also certify and register radiation technologists through education, ethics and examination requirements.

AMERICAN SOCIETY FOR HEALTHCARE ENGINEERING (ASHE)

The national professional organization that represents individuals responsible for the environment of care used in healthcare delivery.

AMERICAN SOCIETY FOR HEALTHCARE RISK MANAGEMENT (ASHRM)

The professional organization for healthcare risk management. Their goal is to advance the risk management profession through professional development, membership services, enhanced communications, risk management innovation and effective governance.

AMERICAN SOCIETY FOR SURGERY OF THE HAND (ASSH)

A professional society of hand surgeons. Their mission is to advance the science and practice of hand and upper extremity surgery through education, research, and advocacy on behalf of patients and practitioners.

AMERICAN SOCIETY HEALTH SYSTEM PHARMACISTS (ASHP)

The professional organization that represents pharmacists who serve as patient care providers in acute and ambulatory settings. The organization's members include pharmacists, student pharmacists and pharmacy technicians. Their mission is to be on the forefront of efforts to improve medication use and enhance patient safety.

AMERICAN SOCIETY OF ANESTHESIOLOGISTS (ASA)

An international educational, research and scientific society that is organized to raise and maintain the standards of the medical practice of anesthesiology. Their mission is to ensure that physician anesthesiologists evaluate and supervise the medical care of patients before, during and after surgery to provide the highest quality and safest care every patient deserves.

AMERICAN SPEECH, LANGUAGE & HEARING ASSOCIATION (ASHA)

A professional, scientific and credentialing association for audiologists, speech–language pathologists, and speech, language, and hearing scientists.

AMERICAN THORACIC SOCIETY (ATS)

An international professional association that was founded in 1905 to combat Tuberculosis and whose mission today is to improve global health by advancing research, patient care, and public health in asthma, COPD, lung cancer, sepsis, acute respiratory distress, and sleep apnea, among other diseases.

ASSOCIATION OF AMERICAN MEDICAL COLLEGES (AAMC)

A non-profit organization that represents the nation's medical schools and teaching hospitals before Congress, federal regulatory agencies, and the executive branch on a wide range of issues. It also administers the Medical College Admission Test which is a computerized examination for prospective students that wish to apply to a medical school in the U.S., Canada and Australia. They also operate the American Medical College Application Service that facilitates students applying to medical schools and the Electronic Residency Application Service through which M.D. and D.O. graduates of medical schools apply to residency and fellowship programs in the U.S.

ASSOCIATION FOR HEALTHCARE RESOURCE AND MATERIALS MANAGEMENT (AHRMM)

The primary organization for healthcare supply chain professionals in the U.S. today. They provide leadership, education, networking, and industry-specific resources to advance their profession and enhance the professional development of its membership. The Association for Healthcare Resource & Materials Management is part of the American Hospital Association.

ASSOCIATION FOR PROFESSIONALS IN INFECTION CONTROL AND EPIDEMIOLOGY, INC. (APIC)

A multi-disciplinary voluntary international organization with over 10,000 members. Its purpose is to influence, support, and improve the quality of healthcare through practicing and managing infection control and applying epidemiology in all healthcare settings. The organization is led by an elected board of members who volunteer their time and expertise.

CENTERS FOR MEDICARE & MEDICAID SERVICES (CMS)

The federal agency in the U.S. Department of Health and Human Services that provides oversight for the Medicare program and works with the states to run the Medicaid program and Children's Health Insurance Programs (CHIP). They determine provider certification and reimbursement. This was formerly called the Health Care Financing Administration or HCFA. They also provide oversight for the Health Insurance Marketplace, and related quality assurance activities.

CLINICAL LABORATORY MANAGERS ASSOCIATION (CLMA)

An association of clinical laboratory professionals that provides support, resources and advocacy in the clinical laboratory industry. They educate and advocate on behalf of their members and play a leadership role in enhancing the image and visibility of the laboratory management profession.

COLLEGE OF AMERICAN PATHOLOGISTS (CAP)

An organization of board-certified pathologists that represents the interests of patients, the public, and pathologists by fostering excellence in the practice of pathology and laboratory medicine worldwide.

COUNCIL OF MEDICAL SPECIALTY SOCIETIES (CMSS)

A non-profit organization that represents the unified voice of forty-one professional societies and 750,000 U.S. physicians formed to discuss issues to improve the United States' healthcare system and health of the public.

DEPARTMENT OF HEALTH AND HUMAN SERVICES (DHHS)

A Federal agency that administers programs for protecting the health and well-being of all Americans by fostering advances in medicine, public health, and social services. They have 11 operating divisions, including eight agencies in the U.S. Public Health Service and three human services agencies.

DRUG ENFORCEMENT ADMINISTRATION (DEA)

The federal agency that licenses individuals to prescribe medications.

FEDERATION OF AMERICAN HOSPITALS (FAH)

A trade association comprised of proprietary or investor-owned hospitals.

FOOD & DRUG ADMINISTRATION (FDA)

The federal agency responsible for protecting the public health by assuring the safety, efficacy and security of drugs, biological products, medical devices, the nation's food supply, and other areas.

FEDERATION OF STATE MEDICAL BOARDS (FSMB)

An organization that represents 70 state medical boards for MDs and DOs within the U.S. Their purpose is to protect the public's health, safety and welfare through the proper licensing, disciplining and regulation of physicians and in most states other healthcare professionals.

HEALTH & HUMAN SERVICES (HHS)

The department that administers all federal programs dealing with health and welfare in the U.S. The agency was started in 1979.

HEALTHCARE FINANCIAL MANAGEMENT ASSOCIATION (HFMA)

The Healthcare Financial Management Association is a non-profit membership organization for healthcare financial management executives. HFMA builds and supports coalitions with other healthcare associations and industry groups to achieve consensus on solutions for the challenges the U.S. healthcare system faces today.

HEALTHCARE INFORMATION AND MANAGEMENT SYSTEMS SOCIETY (HIMSS)

A global, cause-based, not-for-profit organization focused on better health through information technology (IT). HIMSS leads efforts to optimize health engagements and care outcomes using information technology.

HEALTHCARE SUPPLY CHAIN ASSOCIATION (HSCA)

A trade association that represents 14 group purchasing organizations, including for-profit and not-for-profit corporations, purchasing groups, associations, multi-hospital systems and healthcare provider alliances. Their mission is to provide advocacy with all legislative and regulatory authorities, provide education to its members, promote ethical conduct, deliver information and serve as a liaison between health industry organizations engaged in group purchasing and other industry entities on issues of mutual interest.

HEALTH INFORMATION TECHNOLOGY FOR ECONOMIC AND CLINICAL HEALTH (HITECH)

An act within the American Recovery and Reinvestment Act (ARRA) that includes incentives offered to physicians in private practices, as well as institutional practices to implement and adopt electronic medical records. The act also includes a series of fines.

HEALTH INSURANCE PORTABILITY AND ACCOUNTABILITY ACT (HIPAA)

A law designed to improve the efficiency and effectiveness of the nation's health care system, and involves ensuring health insurance coverage, and the privacy and security of health information.

HOSPITAL QUALITY ALLIANCE (HQA)

A collaboration between several national healthcare government and non-profit organizations that was established to promote reporting on hospital quality of care and to share hospital quality information with patients, families, and communities in a unified, consistent manner. The information collected can be viewed on a website called Hospital Compare.

INSTITUTE FOR HEALTHCARE IMPROVEMENT (IHI)

A not-for-profit organization that drives the improvement of healthcare by advancing its quality and value.

INSTITUTE OF MEDICINE (IOM)

An organization within the National Academy of Sciences that acts as an advisor in health and medicine and conducts policy studies relevant to health issues. The IOM is an advisor to federal government on issues of medical care, research, and education.

MEDICAL GROUP MANAGEMENT ASSOCIATION-AMERICAN COLLEGE OF MEDICAL PRACTICE EXECUTIVES (MGMA –ACMPE)

The Medical Group Management Association is a membership association for professional administrators and leaders of medical group practices. In 2011, the MGMA and its standard-setting body, the American College of Medical Practice Executives (ACMPE), voted to merge to form a new association, MGMA-ACMPE. The organization delivers networking, professional education and resources and political advocacy for medical practice management.

NATIONAL ASSOCIATION OF HEALTHCARE TRANSPORT MANAGEMENT (NAHTM)

An educational organization composed of management from the United States and Canada who are responsible for the transportation of patients within hospital settings and which often includes mail services, shuttle/van transportation, equipment management, linen management, distribution, item/materials (including lab specimens) movement, patient lift teams, greeter services, sitter services and volunteer service management.

NATIONAL ASSOCIATION OF HEALTH DATA ORGANIZATIONS (NAHDO)

A non-profit educational association dedicated to improving health care data collection and use. Their members include state and private health data organizations that maintain statewide health care databases and stakeholders of these databases. NAHDO is a cofounder and member of the All Payer Claims Database (APCD) Council, which provides leadership and technical assistance to states implementing APCDs.

NATIONAL ASSOCIATION OF PEDIATRIC NURSE ASSOCIATES/ PRACTITIONERS (NAP-NAP)

A professional association established in 1973 for pediatric nurse practitioners (PNPs) and other advanced practice nurses who provide care for children. Their mission is to improve the quality of health care for infants, children and adolescents, and to promote the PNP's role in providing that care.

NATIONAL BOARD OF MEDICAL EXAMINERS (NBME)

A nonprofit organization responsible for preparing and administering examinations for physicians.

NATIONAL BOARD OF SURGICAL TECHNOLOGY & SURGICAL ASSISTANTS (NBSTSA)

The organization that administers the national certification examination for surgical technologists and surgical assistants. Successful candidates earn the CST or CSFA certification.

NATIONAL CENTER FOR HEALTH STATISTICS (NCHS)

The organization that provides vital statistical information to guide existing and future policies to improve the health of the U.S. population.

NATIONAL COMMITTEE FOR QUALITY ASSURANCE (NCQA)

A national organization that accredits quality assurance programs in prepaid managed care organizations and that assesses the quality of care and service in managed care programs.

NATIONAL COUNCIL OF STATE BOARDS OF NURSING (NCSBN)

An independent, not-for-profit organization through which boards of nursing act (in the 50 states, the District of Columbia and four U.S. territories-Guam, Virgin Islands, American Samoa and the Northern Mariana Islands) and work together on matters of common interest and concern affecting public health, safety and welfare, including the development of nursing licensure examinations.

NATIONAL HEART, LUNG & BLOOD INSTITUTE (NHLBI)

A national organization that promotes the prevention and treatment of heart, lung, and blood diseases by providing global leadership through research, training, and education programs to enhance the health of everyone so that they can live longer and more fulfilling lives.

NATIONAL PATIENT SAFETY GOALS (NPSG)

A program started by the Joint Commission in 2002. They were established to help accredited organizations address specific areas of concern in regard to patient safety issues in a wide variety of health care settings. Each year an advisory group called the Patient Safety Advisory Group meets and advises The Joint Commission on how to address those issues. The Joint Commission also determines whether a goal is applicable to a specific accreditation program and, if so, tailors the goal to be program-specific.

NATIONAL PRACTITIONER DATABANK (NPPB)

An alert or flagging system created to provide a more comprehensive review of professional credentials. It assists state licensing boards, hospitals and other healthcare entities in conducting intensive independent reviews of the qualifications of the healthcare practitioner they seek to license or to grant clinical privileges to. Information reported to the national practitioner data bank is confidential except to those legally allowed to access it.

NATIONAL QUALITY FORUM (NQF)

A private, not-for-profit organization created to develop and implement a national strategy for healthcare quality measurement and reporting.

NATIONAL RURAL HEALTH ASSOCIATION (NHRA)

A nonprofit membership organization whose mission is to provide leadership on rural health issues. Membership consists of a diverse collection of individuals and organizations, all of whom share the common interest in rural healthcare.

NORTH AMERICAN SPINE SOCIETY (NASS)

A multidisciplinary, professional, medical society that utilizes education, research and advocacy to foment the highest quality, ethical, value-and evidence-based spine care for patients throughout the world.

OCCUPATIONAL SAFETY AND HEALTH ADMINISTRATION (OSHA)

An agency of the U. S. Department of Labor charged with the responsibility of reducing occupational exposure and risk to workers' health and safety. OSHA establishes rules, monitors compliance through inspection and enforces rules through penalties and fines for non-compliant organizations.

OFFICE OF THE NATIONAL COORDINATOR OF HEALTH INFORMATION TECHNOLOGY (ONC)

A federal agency within the U.S. Department of Health and Human Services, primarily focused on implementing an interoperable, private and secure nationwide health information system and supporting the widespread, meaningful use of technology. It was founded in 2004 when the medical industry began to incorporate digital record-keeping.

PHYSICIAN CONSORTIUM FOR PERFORMANCE IMPROVEMENT (PCHI)

A national, physician-led program dedicated to enhancing quality and patient safety. The mission of the organization is to align patient-centered care, performance measurement and quality improvement by developing evidence-based performance measures that are clinically meaningful and that are used in national accountability and quality improvement programs.

PHYSICIAN QUALITY REPORTING INITIATIVE (PQRI)

A Medicare program that incentivizes physicians to report data on quality measures by providing bonus payments to participants.

SOCIETY OF CRITICAL CARE MEDICINE (SCCM)

An international, educational and scientific society that was established in 1905 and whose members are health professionals that provide care to critically ill and injured patients. In addition to research and education the Society is also an advocate on issues related to critical care.

APPENDIX 4

Prescription Terms—Administration Methods—Frequency

Bol - Bolus	prn - As Needed
a.c. - Before Meals	O.S. - In the Left Eye
I.M - Intramuscularly	q.d - Every Day
a.m. - Morning before Noon	O.U. - In Both Eyes
Inj - Injection	q.h. - Every Hour
b.i.d. - Twice per Day	p.o.- Orally
GM, gm, G- Gram	q.h.s - Before Bed
IP - Intraperitoneal	Rectally-Rectally
dc/disc - Discontinue	q.i.d. - Four Times a Day
I.V. - Intravenous	Subq.- Subcutaneous
Noc - Nocturnal	q.o.d. - Every Other Hour
IVP - Intravenous Push	Tab - Tablet
p.c. - After Meals	q.t.t. - Drop
IVPB - Intravenous Piggyback	q.4h - Every Four Hours
p.m. - Afternoon, Evening	q.6h - Every Six Hours
O.D. - In the Right Eye	5X a day - Five Times a Day

ABOUT THE AUTHORS

Tom Williams is a former senior executive with general management and sales and marketing expertise with major health care organizations. For 25 years he consistently built shareholder value by selling and marketing high technology products and services in the domestic and international markets.

His background as a Vice President of Sales & Marketing includes selling high technology medical products and services through a variety of distribution channels in a wide array of markets. He was also the CEO of two specialty hospitals, the Vice President & General Manager of an ancillary services division and the President of a medical services company.

Tom's personal profile includes a bachelor's degree in biology from the University of Detroit. He has a Master's degree in Management (MAM) and a Master's degree in Business (MBA) from the Peter F. Drucker and Masatoshi Ito Graduate School of Management at Claremont Graduate University. He is also a registered and certified respiratory therapist. Strategic Dynamics publishes a weekly Healthcare Business Acumen & Sales Insights blog, several E-Books and a Healthcare Insights Series. He resides in Scottsdale, AZ.

Heather L. Williams is a former sales professional that sold complex medical equipment into the Operating Rooms of hospitals and surgery centers. After a successful sales career she joined Strategic Dynamics.

In her current role she is responsible for the company website, blog and all other media produced by the company. She also handles most of the market research projects and sells and delivers consulting around the Everything DISC® Profiles to clients.

Heather is a graduate from Arizona State University with a Bachelor of Science (B.S.) in Business Administration. She resides in Phoenix, Arizona.

ABOUT STRATEGIC DYNAMICS

We help organizations execute their vision and drive results by providing insight, process and tools to improve sales performance. Our specialty is the healthcare continuum.

We offer a wide array of consulting services and training programs that deliver measurable results. Our foundation program is entitled "Selling Within Hospitals: Business Acumen." This customizable program teaches the function and operation of a hospital with or without a sales simulation. It's unique because it has been designed by hospital CEOs.

To help improve sales skills we represent a wide array of products, services and tools through MHI Global. To help sales professionals improve their communication and selling style we offer the Everything DISC® Sales Profile.

For the past 15 years Strategic Dynamics has worked with medical device start-ups to global organizations. We have also managed hospitals and worked with hospital management organizations. We understand GPOs, IDNs, RPCs and distributors. Call for a free consultation to see if we can help you.